HOW TO
LIVE
UNTIL YOU DIE

The 7 Keys to Living
Happy, Healthy & Whole

To Tom & Debbie,

May You Live Really Live!

Prob. 4:22 MSG

THANK YOU!

I've created an additional resource I want you
to have as a thank you for your purchase,
so get it now by visiting:

HowToLiveUntilYouDie.com/thanks

*"Dear friend, I pray that you may enjoy good
health and that all may go well with you,
even as your soul is getting along well."*
– 3 John 1:2 (NIV)

Praise for *How to Live Until You Die*

Finally, here's a return to common sense and a call to intelligent simplicity in the area of our health. No fad diets, no exotic exercise plans, no expensive gurus, no fancy equipment, no cookie-cutter approach, but a gentle encouragement to nurture the simple requirements of our body, mind and spirit. I've experienced the life-changing benefits of trusting this pharmacist who is telling us to stop buying the medications he was taught to sell, and start living a restful, stress-free, and abundant life.

Dan Miller
Author and Coach
48Days.com

Dr. Phil Carson's devotion to help others in their journey to find and maintain a healthier lifestyle shines through in this practical, easy-to-read book. How To Live Until You Die *is an excellent mixture of science, personal stories, and practical recommendations that provides a clear roadmap to improving your health. Having known Dr. Carson for many years, I have learned that he possesses a unique skill of softly instructing, encouraging, and entertaining people in their journey to optimal wellness.*

Dr. Allison Ford-Wade, Ph.D.
Associate Professor of Health Promotion
Director, Bone Density Laboratory
Department of Health,
Exercise Science and Recreation Management
The University of Mississippi

If you are like me, you don't want to take another pill to avoid death. We want to make decisions to live fully for as long as possible. Dr. Phil provides the common sense guide to enable each of us to make the decision for a better today and more tomorrows. I most highly recommend this encouraging and actionable book.

Tom Schwab
Founder of Interview Valet

I'm an entrepreneur who has experienced life to its fullest in many areas except health. I honestly felt terrible physically until I met Dr. Phil Carson. I didn't know or understand the negative consequences of many prescriptions, inactivity, and bad food choices. What an amazing transformation I've experienced with such minimal adjustments. Dr. Phil has revolutionized the way I think, which allows me to truly live until I die. I feel a sense of gratitude that I can't explain. I'm now living a life of complete abundance emotionally, spiritually, and physically.

Aaron Walker
View from the Top
Premier Life/Business Coach & Author

Every person I know wants to maximize and extend each day of their life. Dr Carson's prescription for living fully alive brings health to every area of living. I have personally benefited from his wisdom and recommend How to Live Until You Die.

Ken Davis
Speaker
Comedian
Author of *Fully Alive*
Founder of Dynamic Communicators International

In a culture and world that worships health and vitality, and is saturated with quick fixes, miracle pills, and the promises of overnight success, it is refreshing to know, that the truth, is alive and well. With 30 years pharmaceutical experience, Dr. Carson lays out seven, must-know pieces to the health and wellness puzzle. Don't read this book. Study it.

Joel Boggess
Speaker, Podcaster, and Author of *Finding Your Voice*

HOW TO
LIVE
UNTIL YOU DIE

The 7 Keys to Living
Happy, Healthy & Whole

Dr. Phil Carson

ISBN-13: 978-0-9984742-0-5

Edited by Jennifer Harshman, HarshmanServices.com
Cover by Rebecca McKeever
Book Design by James Woosley, FreeAgentPress.com

To Kim, my beautiful wife.

Kim, your love and support for me over the years has been more than I could have ever dreamed of or asked for. You've been an amazing wife and wonderful mother to our five children. I know you'll be a wonderful grandmother to Charlee and all our future grands as well.

Thank you for all you've done to make our home the kind of home I always dreamed of.

Your love and support makes it possible for me to live happy, healthy and whole.

DISCLAIMER

CONTENTS

ACKNOWLEDGMENTS

This book would not have been possible without the unwavering support and encouragement of many people.

Thank you to my kids, Cody, Clay, Anna Kathryn, Claire, and Caroline for believing in me, even as I struggled to teach you right and be the best Dad I could be.

Thank you to Dan Miller for your friendship, mentorship, and inspiration, which helped me believe more in myself and my abilities, so I could accomplish more than I ever dreamed I could.

Thank you to Andy Traub for helping me pull all the parts together to make this book a reality. Thank you for your guidance, coaching, and pushing me to get it done.

Thank you to the gifted and talented Nick Pavlidis who helped me turn all the information and stories I had accumulated over the decades into the book you're about to read.

Thank you to Aaron Walker for your constant encouragement and coaching me through some difficult and trying days prior to and during the writing of this book.

Thank you to Jeff McMahon for your contributions to the exercise chapter and for helping me become more physically fit than I've been in 30 years.

Thank you to all the members of my mastermind group who've inspired and encouraged me through this process.

Thank you to all the clients that I have had the opportunity to serve over the years. You've made my life so much more rewarding.

Thank you to Rebecca McKeever, Jennifer Harshman, and James Woosley for your incredible design, editing, layout, and production contributions. Your talents have transformed words on a screen to a book that has the potential to help people around the world.

Thank you to my Heavenly Father, for always listening to me, walking with me and sometimes carrying me. Thank you Father for breathing into my spirit the words, I am happy, I am healthy, I am whole. Without you I wouldn't be any of the three.

INTRODUCTION

"There are two obstacles to vibrant health and longevity: ignorance and complacency."

– World Health Organization

WHAT IF **I** COULD show you seven areas of your life that have been proven to work together to lead to better mental, emotional, and physical health, no matter what your past looks like or how old you are?

What if I also could show you simple, natural, and effective ways to improve each of those areas without requiring you to spend thousands of dollars or spend hours working through some complicated "system"?

And, finally, what if I told you that by implementing the simple and effective concepts, you can not only live a healthier and more vibrant, feeling good life for yourself, but you could also change your family tree, improving the lives of the people you love the most, as well as future generations of your family?

Well, it's all true.

"The purpose of life is not to be happy. It is to be useful, to be honorable, to be compassionate, to have it make some difference that you have lived and lived well."
– Ralph Waldo Emerson

We live in a time where stress levels are higher than ever; work, family, and community demands are stronger than ever; and tending to ourselves is sometimes viewed as selfish or worse by the discriminating eyes of people who

are so stressed and depressed themselves that the
other people down in an effort to find comfort. We'r
feeling stressed, tired, depressed, imbalanced, and lost. We
feel out of control and like our spouses, kids, colleagues,
bosses, and others all have more control over our health,
wealth, and well-being than we do.

It doesn't have to be that way. We're all three-part
beings consisting of body, soul, and spirit, and we need to
nurture all three of those parts to be whole and be effective at home and at work. We need to be physically, mentally, and emotionally healthy. We need to take control.
You need to take control, and I can help.

You don't need some complicated system. You don't
need to start over, or go back in time. You don't need to
add three more hours to your day or sleep four hours a
night (In fact, I'll show you why that can actually hurt you
physically, mentally, and emotionally!). You don't need to
spend thousands of dollars.

You can start right where you are, right now, and live
a happier, healthier, and more whole life, and I can give
you the information, inspiration, and will to tap into the
power you already have within you.

You can start living an extraordinary life—today—by
making simple changes in just seven key areas of your
life, which you can easily remember through the acronym N.E.W.S.S.S.S., which stands for Nutrition, Exercise, Water, Sleep, Supplements, Soul, and Spirit. Those

seven areas of life are your seven keys to becoming happy, healthy, and whole. You hold all seven of those keys. This book is designed to help give you information and inspiration to attend to those seven key areas plus simple, practical ways to incorporate healthy habits into your daily life in each of the areas. With this information and inspiration, and these practical tips, you can work with your local health-care providers to implement a balanced and simple but effective plan that is custom designed for your unique needs to improve your mental, emotional, and physical health. This plan addresses each of the seven key N.E.W.S.S.S.S. areas of your life.

> *"The key to keeping your balance is knowing when you've lost it."*
> **– Anonymous**

I have worked with thousands of people just like you, for over three decades, to help them become happy, healthy, and whole by making simple shifts to their nutrition, exercise, water intake, supplement consumption, sleep patterns, spiritual life, and connectedness to their inner souls.

I've discovered the biggest obstacle for many people wasn't a lack of information about these key areas, but that there's too much information—and a lot of misinformation—about these areas, causing people to freeze and get overwhelmed. The result was that too many people were improving one or two areas temporarily but couldn't stick with it or improve other important areas because it was too complicated, expensive, or disruptive to their lifestyle.

Nutrition became subscribing to having a monthly box of powder sent to your house, or drinking a shake for two meals a day, or forcing any number of specialty diets into your life. Exercise became expensive, complicated, or extreme programs that cost a lot of money, take a lot of time, or require you to be someone you aren't. Water consumption became a chore. Supplements became expensive or too processed and ineffective. Sleep became "for the weak." Soul searching became something only Millennials did when they didn't want to get a "real job." And spirituality became taboo or associated with only one way of thinking.

The confusion and commercialism associated with these seven areas caused the terms to essentially become curse words, calling up feelings that remind us that we are unhealthy or unhappy.

Nobody would want to "exercise" if it meant they had to flip tires, hang from a hula hoop tied to the ceiling, or jump up and down on a trampoline for an hour.

And how many times have you heard someone at work brag because they consistently get the right amount of sleep? These days, sleeping less carries a dangerous badge of honor.

These are just two examples of how too much information and misinformation have led people into living a less healthy, more imbalanced lifestyle.

As I worked with more people, I realized that there was no single, reliable resource that provided easy-to-implement solutions while addressing the misinformation in all seven key areas in a way that is simple yet comprehensive.

People came to me for answers, and I'd have to pull answers from dozens, if not hundreds of places, synthesize the information for them, and then guide them as they made better, more informed decisions about their health.

I became determined to make that into one resource, which you are now reading, so that you can cut through the chaos of biased advice, misinformation, and piecemeal support, and live a happy, healthy, and whole life.

In pulling this together, I have identified simple, research-based solutions for each of these areas. I give you both the "how" and the "why" it is critical that you work in these key areas. And most importantly, I make it easy for you to apply it to your lifestyle.

Where did it all start?

My research for this book started in 1979, at the University of Mississippi School of Pharmacy, from where I graduated with a Bachelors of Science in Pharmacy. After six years of intense study, I earned my pharmacy degree in 1985, and immediately began working in a local pharmacy.

Since that time, I have become certified as a compounding pharmacist, a diabetes care pharmacist, and, most recently, a consulting pharmacist.

With all that traditional education, you might think that I am just another voice for traditional medicine, but that couldn't be further from the truth. From an early stage in my career, I observed several significant gaps in mental, emotional, and physical health that traditional medicine either couldn't or wouldn't address. I grew frustrated as countless clients and customers came into the pharmacy to pick up a traditional solution that only temporarily masked the symptoms of their condition and did nothing to address the underlying condition that caused the symptoms to begin with.

From unhealthy weight-loss pills, to diabetes medications, to attention-support drugs and many more, clients came to me with a prescription that they thought solved their problems, but in reality did nothing of the sort.

After a few years of observing these struggles, I started learning as much as I could about natural and alternative remedies. I searched for help with the underlying causes or conditions and not just a pill that would help people lose a few pounds, concentrate for a few hours, or feel numb for a day or two.

In doing so, I received numerous certifications in natural and alternative medicine therapies, so I could learn new and natural ways to help people, and became certified as a lifestyle coach and 48 Days Certified Coach so I could identify solutions that people could actually apply to their lives and learn how to best guide people to making more informed choices about their health and continue to support them into the future.

I didn't just learn about these remedies., I started offering them as alternative solutions and used my lifestyle and 48 Days coaching training to make sure these solutions were simple, practical, and effective enough for people to benefit from them over the long term.

> *"Let us endeavor to live so that when we die even the undertaker will be sorry."*
> **– Mark Twain**

The more I learned about these solutions, and the more people I helped, the more I began to believe that natural and alternative solutions play an important role—in addition to traditional pharmaceutical remedies and non-medicinal activities—in forming a well-rounded mental, emotional, and physical health plan.

I firmly believe that the traditional way of healthcare is not sustainable and the future of healthcare is in identifying and treating the causes of disease, not just masking or treating symptoms.

As Thomas Edison once famously said, "The doctor of the future will give no medicine, but will interest his patients in the care of the human body, in diet, and in the cause and prevention of disease."

Although Edison's prediction occurred a long time ago, I'm beginning to see his prediction coming true, as more healthcare professionals are shifting their approaches and more consumers are educated and demanding real cures.

How important are these seven areas? Look at what improving in these areas did for Sam.

If you looked at Sam today, you would see someone who is full of joy, happy and healthy. He's married to a wonderful woman, has well-adjusted kids, is at the top of his career, and lives in his dream house. He has everything he needs and a lot of what he wants.

But life wasn't always so great for Sam. During his formative years, Sam lived in the Deep South in a house full of turmoil, fear, substandard nutrition, physical abuse, and inconsistent spiritual and emotional well-being.

Sam's father struggled for most of his adult life. He had an inconsistent relationship with his own father, at best, although Sam didn't know why. His father was also angry much of the time and took his out anger on Sam, his brother, and his mother.

Sam lived in constant fear and anxiety. He walked on eggshells because his father was so violent and unpredictable. Sometimes, something he said would set his father off. Other times, it was something he did. Sometimes, it was nothing. His father just woke up or came home upset and went off on everyone.

After a number of attempts to change, his father finally sought help and things at home stabilized. His anger was under control. His mood swings subsided. And he even started reading the Bible, going to church, and preaching. He seemed to be pulling his life together. Although they didn't know it at the time, his father would later reveal that he had an encounter with God and it made him a different, better person. He began to feel worthy and connected to a bigger purpose.

After that encounter, Sam's dad stabilized for a short period of time. He'd frequently sit on the patio reading his Bible. He was calm. He was kind. He was supportive. He was everything Sam ever wanted in a father, until one morning at church, a church deacon told him they made a mistake by allowing him to preach and he wouldn't be allowed to preach anymore. He was crushed. His newfound meaning was shattered. He no longer felt connected to that greater purpose. And he immediately regressed.

Sam couldn't stand being home and avoided it as much as he could. He didn't feel safe. He didn't feel important. He didn't feel loved. He never had a friend visit or sleep over out of fear of what might happen with his father.

The only thing that saved him was the support of two loving grandmothers, who lived close by. They were strong women with a deep Christian faith who loved Sam well. They were a tremendous influence. After school, on weekends, and throughout the summer, Sam spent as much time with his grandmothers as he could, and even spent every summer for the first seven or eight years of school with them.

Sleeping at his grandmother's house was peaceful. He didn't have to worry that something he said or did would get him or his mother beat. They fed him well, took him to church, read the Bible to him, and had him read the Bible to them. They sat for hours, talking and putting puzzles together. He ate well, slept better, and got to be a kid without fear.

When he was thirteen, he even started going to church on his own, and then with a friend. He, too, had an encounter with God and found healthy men through the church who mentored him and showed him what it was like to be a good man. His youth minister was incredible, too. Sam started feeling connected to something bigger than himself.

Sam also started playing football and found a great mentor in his football coach, who told him he was proud of him. He felt love and stability.

The effect of the instability lasted long after Sam moved out and Sam recalls struggling to feel truly fulfilled or happy for the first twenty-six years of his life. Even after he married an incredibly strong woman, he still held on to the pain from his childhood. Only after they welcomed their first child, at twenty-seven years old, with a happy marriage, beautiful child, and a strong career, did Sam feel more whole on a consistent basis.

What changed for Sam?

What changed by the time his first kid was born? Everything.

As a child, he ate processed, unhealthy food, lacked exercise and activity, slept lightly, took no supplements, struggled with a wounded soul, and experienced only inconsistent spiritual enlightenment. As he got older, he found help, started working out, played sports, and ate better. He also started mentoring and ministering to younger kids as he grew spiritually.

After he got married, he found new purpose with his wife, made better choices, and experienced success in his profession. He was less stressed, continued to eat and sleep better, and had a healthy spiritual life. When his son was born, he felt an even deeper meaning to life. He felt important, responsible, and connected to a bigger purpose.

What about those people who aren't as broken as Sam was?

Sam's story is extreme. He went from deficient in all seven N.E.W.S.S.S.S. key areas to happy, healthy, and whole. He took all seven areas from deficient to full.

Most people aren't deficient in all seven areas, however, and only need to improve in a few of them to live a healthy, vibrant, feeling good life. For those people, the "N.E.W.S.S.S.S." is good because as simple as it is to improve all seven areas, it is that much easier to only need to improve one or two areas.

In fact, some people can unlock true health and happiness by becoming more informed and making different choices in just one area, like Jerry.

Lacking in one area can make an enormous difference.

Jerry's wife walked into my pharmacy with a prescription in hand. I had just started learning about natural medicine at the time and still worked almost exclusively with traditional pharmaceuticals. I may have had two or three natural medicine certification courses under my belt at that point and was running my first pharmacy in a small town called Smithville, Mississippi.

This was her first time in my pharmacy, so after I filled her prescription, I walked around the counter to let her know about the side effects. Midway through, she confided in me that her husband was in hospice care and was sent home to die. He had end-stage congestive heart failure and wasn't expected to live long.

Although I only had two or three natural medicine certification courses under my belt at the time, one of them was on heart health from a course taught by a cardiologist from Johns Hopkins Hospital. In that course, I learned about Coenzyme Q10, or CoQ10, something our bodies naturally produce, although in lesser quantities as we age. CoQ10, I learned, naturally energizes our muscles, including heart muscles, which was why the instructor said he gave it to all of his heart patients. Because we produce less CoQ10 as we age, supplementing it naturally can make a big difference, I learned.

Because I knew from my pharmaceutical experience that when people are prescribed statin drugs, they commonly experience muscle weakness, it occurred to me that CoQ10 could naturally combat that common side effect by reenergizing those muscles. And because millions of people take statin drugs, I bought some CoQ10 for my pharmacy right after taking that course.

Everything she told me about Jerry made me feel that CoQ10 had a chance to help him, too, so I told her there might be a natural supplement that could help and encouraged her to consider giving some to Jerry. She was a nurse who was off from work to care for Jerry until he passed, and hadn't heard of CoQ10. She was curious, though, and said she would talk to his doctor about whether it was worth a shot.

The next day, she returned. She and the doctor had researched CoQ10. In her words, the doctor said it "couldn't hurt" and suggested a specific dosage to "see what happens," because Jerry was going to die anyway. She thanked me for my suggestion, bought a bottle, and left.

A couple of weeks later, she returned and asked to talk with me. She was in tears. I feared the worst.

"I wish I had taken pictures for you to see the difference in Jerry," she said. "He was swollen almost twice his normal size. He couldn't even get out of bed to go to the bathroom. He's back to his normal size and able to get out of bed to go to the bathroom on his own. I need another bottle of CoQ10."

Retaining water, or edema, is common with congestive heart failure. It was no surprise that Jerry had been swollen, but the changes he experienced in just two weeks were miraculous. We talked for a few more minutes about the progress Jerry had made so quickly. By the end of the conversation, we were both in tears.

Another month brought another miracle.

A month or so later, Jerry's wife returned. This time she was smiling. After another month of CoQ10, Jerry got out of the house and to Walmart. "Although I brought him in on a wheelchair," she explained, "when we got in the store, he got up and walked around on his own."

Less than two months earlier, he was sent home to die. Now he was walking around Walmart with his wife.

As the months went by, the miracles continued. On her next visit, she told me Jerry had mowed the back lawn and would have mowed the front lawn, too, but he was supposed to have been dead and didn't want people to see him so active. A few months later, he returned to work as a truck driver.

The visits stopped.

After about six months or so, she stopped coming in. I had no idea what happened. I hoped and prayed they moved away or found another pharmacy, but feared that his heart condition worsened and he passed away. I thought about them often.

A year or two later, she returned out of the blue. The moment I saw her, I dropped everything and came around the counter.

"It's so great to see you. I haven't seen you in so long. How have you been?" I asked. I feared her response.

"We moved away, but I was in the neighborhood and wanted to come by to see you," she responded, choking up a bit. My heart sank into my stomach.

"Jerry passed away," she said.

"I'm so sorry," I said. "What happened?"

"It wasn't his heart. That's why I wanted to stop in. He had a rare liver disease that went undetected and it killed him. His heart was fine and I just wanted to stop by today and thank you. Thank you for telling me about CoQ10.

Thank you for what you did for Jerry and me. Over the past two years, Jerry went from bedridden, dejected, and ready to die, to even better than before. In fact, before he died, he got his life right with God and I know he's in heaven. So thank you for everything."

As a young pharmacist who had an encounter with God that changed my life, that last part touched me deeply. On top of that, the fact that better-informed health care and a natural option helped someone like Jerry so deeply made me more determined than ever to learn even more about natural medicines and supplements. It lit a fire in me that burns brighter every day.

Since that time, I have helped thousands of people make positive changes in their lives by helping them work on whatever parts of the N.E.W.S.S.S.S. key areas of life they struggle with. Whether you struggle in all seven areas like Sam did, or just need a new perspective and information in just one or two areas like Jerry did, new perspectives and progress in these seven areas can help you live a happier, more vibrant, feeling good life.

Over the next seven chapters, I will show you exactly how—and why—each of these areas can help you. We will work our way right through the N.E.W.S.S.S.S. acronym from Nutrition, to Exercise, to Water, to Sleep, to Supplements, to Soul, and Spirit.

For each of these key areas of life, I will give you the science behind why they are so important to your well-being, as well as simple, practical ways for you to start living a happier, healthier life.

No matter what your past or present looks like, if you take the information I am about to share with you, and you work with your family and professionals to apply them in your life, your future can be happy, healthy, and whole.

CHAPTER 1
NUTRITION

How to Stop Dieting, Toss the Diet Pills,
and Start Eating Well on a Budget

*"If the doctors of today do not become
the nutritionists of tomorrow,
then the nutritionists of today
will become the doctors of tomorrow."*

– Rockefeller Institute of Medical Research

WITH ALL THE PULLS on our time and money these days, it's no wonder so many people are stressed out and struggling to eat healthfully. Years of stress-induced emotional eating,[1] quick trips through a dangerous fast-food drive through, and conflicting information about healthy eating have left too many people unhealthy, demoralized, and tired. In fact, according to the United States Center for Health Statistics, over 70% of adults over twenty years old are overweight or obese.[2]

The risks of being overweight or obese are extraordinary and include diabetes, heart disease, high blood pressure, fatty liver disease, osteoarthritis, stroke, sleep apnea, gallstones, and even some types of cancer.[3] Given the number of Americans who are overweight and the grave risks associated with that, it's easy to see how the weight-loss industry has grown into a multi-billion-dollar industry.

> *"1/4 of what you eat keeps you alive… 3/4 of what you eat keeps your doctor alive."*
> **– Dr. Andrew Saul**

Fad diets, weight-loss pills, and invasive weight-loss surgeries are just three parts of a largely unregulated industry that has caused people to believe that they have only three options when it comes to eating and weight management: (1) spend a lot of time and money popping pills and adjusting their lifestyle to fit a complicated diet of expensive, bland food, (2) spending thousands of dollars on highly invasive surgeries, or (3) eating unhealthy foods that are convenient, cheap, and taste good but are full of toxins and can make them overweight and unhealthy.

Every year people spend billions of dollars chasing a miracle cure to their weight problem only to find out that there is no miracle.

Even worse, there's so much contradictory information being spread that it's difficult to know what to believe about healthy eating. One day we're told to avoid fat. Later we find out that not all fat is bad, only some fat. Later we're told to avoid carbohydrates. Later still, we find out that only some, but not all, carbohydrates are bad.

From a medicinal side, weight-loss pills have become a multi-billion-dollar industry, with advertisement upon advertisement touting the next "miracle pill" that will help you burn fat, suppress your appetite, speed up your metabolism, or block your body from absorbing fat or carbohydrates. When you dig deep behind the claims, however, you'll find many of the supposed miracles are dangerous and ineffective. In fact, the United States Federal Trade Commission has found so many lies and so much exaggeration in advertising claims for weight-loss products and services that they warn consumers right on their website that those claims "inherently over-promise"[4] and warn that claims that you can eat all you want and still lose weight effortlessly because of some miracle pill "just aren't true."[5] Yet every year people spend billions of dollars chasing a miracle cure to their weight problem only to find out that there is no miracle.

Finally, some people go to even more extreme measures to lose weight, like invasive surgeries to change the anatomy or function of their digestive systems. Although some of these methods can be effective in extreme circumstances under the careful advice and supervision of a trained professional, invasive surgeries are not always effective over the long term and can be extremely dangerous. In fact, a 2010 study of patients who underwent gastric bypass surgery found that 41% of patients hadn't lost any weight and 51% demonstrated behavior consistent with eating disorders.[6]

Because of all this misinformation and all this confusion, people end up bouncing from fad diet to fad diet, from "miracle pill" to "miracle pill," or just give up altogether. They end up stressed, dejected, depressed, and guilt-ridden. They continue to function with low energy and decreased mental functionality, and stay on a path to potentially devastating long-term health consequences.

I've been there, too.

When I was a young pharmacist with a young family, I too fell into bad eating habits and got caught up in a fad diet. I had tried my best to eat healthfully, but thought it had to be complicated and time consuming, and with a busy job and young family who needed my time, too, I turned to the hot fad diet at the time: the fat-free diet. Although I initially lost weight, I soon realized that the benefits were narrow and temporary.

In my professional and personal lives, I've also witnessed people with bags of pills they had bought to help them lose weight, only to find out that they didn't work or caused severe side effects. I listened as they told me they bought the pills because they thought the pills were a simple option, although none of them really knew what they were putting into their bodies. They saw an advertisement on TV or the internet, or heard from a friend that the pills would help them lose weight and that's all they needed to buy the pills and start taking them.

Any successful nutrition plan has four requirements.

In order for a nutrition plan to work over the long term, it must be proven to work safely over the long term, offer a balanced solution that allows you to eat a variety of foods and not require you to deprive yourself of entire categories of food, and be flexible enough to work with your lifestyle and budget. If any of those are missing, you'll be setting yourself up for failure from the start. That's exactly why most fad diets and miracle pills don't work over the long term.

> *"People are fed by the food industry, which pays no attention to health, and are treated by the health industry, which pays no attention to food."*
> **– Wendell Berry**

First, most diets aren't about you. They aren't made to fit *your* lifestyle. They force you to adjust your life to fit their rules. Of course, not all of that is bad. If your typical breakfast includes a jelly-filled donut and a milkshake with a splash of coffee, even I would tell you it's time to adjust. But too many diets require you to adjust everything about what you eat. Not only is that a problem from a lifestyle perspective, it leaves you set up to fail. This often leads to people doubting their ability to improve their health and leaves them one small failure away from slipping right back into unhealthy habits.

Second, many diets and miracle pills are expensive. Diets that make you buy special food or powders, or pay to be a member or per pound lost can get expensive. Miracle pills often rope you into a subscription, up-sells, and recurring charges that can add up to hundreds or thousands of dollars per year.

Third, too many diets are about unhealthy deprivation, not healthy balance. "Next to love, balance is the most important thing." Those famous words were spoken by the great John Wooden. Although many people apply those outside of the nutritional world, they apply equally well to how you eat. Too many diets tell you to throw the baby out with the bath water, telling you to eliminate all fats or carbohydrates, when only some fats are unhealthy and when eliminating or greatly limiting *only* the unhealthy ones is both simple and beneficial. Worse yet, some diets ask you to skip entire meals on a regular basis or replace real food with their own frozen or canned options, or worse, powders, which are often full of dangerous toxins that are found in the very foods that are making you sick, tired, and overweight to begin with.

Finally, most diets and miracle pills aren't proven to work over the long term. In fact, they're often designed to work quickly, leading to quick fixes and a false sense of accomplishment after seeing weight that took years to gain drop in a matter of weeks.

There is another option.

There *is* another option, though—a better plan— that anyone can use to eat convenient, healthy food that tastes good. This option is cost effective and simple. It is quick and easy. It's about balance. It doesn't require any "miracles," and it can fit into anyone's budget and lifestyle. I'll give you this third option in this chapter.

This option will help you forget about fad diets and begin incorporating balanced, healthy eating habits into your life, which will serve you well for the long term. This plan is simple and effective enough to help you make better eating choices no matter where you are, what your family and friends choose to eat, or what your food budget is.

> *The problem is not so simple*
> *as merely cutting down or*
> *eliminating sugars and white flour,*
> *though this is exceedingly important.*
> *It is also necessary that*
> *adequate mineral and vitamin*
> *carrying foods be made available."*
> **– Dr. Weston A. Price**

This plan will help you feel better about eating well, give you increased productivity, control blood sugar levels for more sustained energy, and elevate your mood and mental clarity. All of these benefits can be yours without breaking your budget, completely flipping your lifestyle, or putting an unknown mix of chemicals into your body.

This plan is an important piece of the overall health

plan that I cover in this book, walking you through the seven N.E.W.S.S.S.S. key areas that anyone can use to be more healthy, happy, and whole. Together with the other six N.E.W.S.S.S.S. key areas, this plan will help you avoid falling into the trap of wasting time and money on ineffective, extreme, and potentially dangerous or ineffective fad diets or "miracle pills."

Try a better, natural plan.

Any plan that is built to succeed must work with your lifestyle to ensure you can and will keep up with it. It must be simple and allow you to eat real food that fits within your budget so you can stick with it at work, at home, and even in restaurants. It must be about balance, so you can have a variety of food and nutrients. Finally, it must be sustainable and proven to work over the long term.

If you're looking to improve your overall health in a way that allows you to eat real food that tastes good and can fit in your lifestyle and budget, I have a better plan. This plan is about balance. It's about avoiding the foods that have been proven to contain dangerous toxins or cause disease or weight gain and replacing them with healthy food that tastes good and fits into *your* lifestyle and budget. It's about making simple choices on a daily basis and is built on a simple five-step framework to eating clean and healthy foods.

Step 1: Avoid the Big Seven Toxins.

Artificial sweeteners: aspartame (always avoid), sucralose (the lesser of two evils to aspartame), saccharin (Sweet'N Low®)

- High fructose corn syrup

- Trans fats, hydrogenated oils such as margarine and shortening. Many peanut butters are actually trans fats.

- Artificial flavorings: can cause problems, especially with hyperactive, ADHD, autistic kids.

- Monosodium glutamate (MSG): causes all kinds of neurological problems. Dr. Russell Blalock calls it an excitotoxin—excites the nervous system. Neurotoxic chemical.

- Artificial colors: Red 40, Blue 1, etc., can cause problems, especially with hyperactive, ADHD, autistic kids. It can ramp them up.

- Preservatives to keep food from spoiling: two in particular are in processed foods: BHT and BHA, butilated chemicals. BHT is found in a lot of nutritional products like multivitamins, as a preservative. Toluene (BHT) is a chemical that is used in dry cleaning clothes. BHA has been shown to cause cancer.

Fortunately it is relatively easy to avoid these because they're found mostly in processed foods. By eliminating or at least minimizing processed and fast foods, you can be confident that you're eliminating many of these Big Seven Toxins.

Fast food, in particular, has become more popular as lives have become busier. This is a very troubling trend that can have incredibly harmful results on our health if we don't begin to make wise choices. For example, a fifteen-year study of over 3,000 people found "Fast-food consumption has strong positive associations with weight gain and insulin resistance, suggesting that fast food increases the risk of obesity and Type 2 diabetes."[7] Beyond these health effects, if you take a quick scan of the ingredients in fast food, you will find instance after instance of preservatives, artificial flavors and colors, and more of the Big Seven Toxins.[8]

If you do end up at a fast-food restaurant, go for a salad and skip the creamy dressings. It won't be the healthiest or tastiest salad in your life, but it will help you avoid many of the Big Seven Toxins until your next scheduled healthy snack or clean meal, and it's much better than the fried foods or sandwiches.

Step 2: Know what to eat and how to find it.

1. Read the labels, especially if you're buying anything in a box. Watch for the Big Seven Toxins. Avoid them—especially the cereal aisle! On a recent trip to the grocery store, I read the labels on nearly every cereal in the aisle. I found at least two of the Big Seven Toxins on every label I read. In fact, one breakfast food had all seven.

2. Identify restaurants ahead of time that serve clean food, so you're not in a rush to make a choice in a pinch. Get salads. Use olive oil and vinegar for dressing, or squeezed lemon.

3. Spend more time in the produce department and less time in the cereal and bread aisles. Fresh food is best. Fresh frozen is okay, too, if you need it to last a bit.

4. Focus on more balanced eating. Stop depriving yourself of entire categories. Balance your meals properly. We have three major macronutrients: protein, carbohydrates, and fat. You need to get some of each of these almost every time you eat.

   - **Protein:** Protein is important to help you control your blood sugar. It is important that you have protein during each meal. Examples of good protein sources are fish, chicken, beef, and eggs.

   - **Carbohydrates:** Carbohydrates are an important source of energy. It's important to focus on good sources of carbohydrates, however, because some carbohydrates cause your blood sugar to spike, which can cause weight gain in the long term and your energy levels to go up and down in the short term. I suggest most people get their carbohydrates from low-glycemic fruits and vegetables. Those are generally the best ways to get natural, healthy carbohydrates. If you go beyond fruits and vegetables, whole grains are a next-best choice because, although they can cause weight gain if consumed in large quantities, they generally maintain the vitamins, minerals, fiber, and other key nutrients that other, simple-carbohydrate sources don't. Simple carbohydrates generally lack essential nutrients and can cause energy crashes and weight gains. For those reasons, I suggest most people severely reduce or even eliminate simple carbohydrates from their diets. Examples of simple carbohydrates include white foods like processed flour, sugar, dairy, and white potatoes.

- **Fat:** We need fats. Our bodies can't live without them. But there are good fats and bad fats. My focus with the clients I advise is to eliminate bad fats from their diets, which include trans fats like margarine, for example, and replace them with healthy, good fats. Examples of good fats include most nuts, real butter (in moderation), olive oil, fish oil, avocado, and coconut oil.

Balance those three every time you're eating and you'll be well on your way to a healthier nutritional lifestyle.

Here's a simple way to estimate the balance between protein, good carbohydrates, and good fats so you can achieve a more balanced and healthy eating plan without having to weigh everything you eat: Imagine you're eating a meal on one of those white plastic plates that are divided into three sections. Whether you have a sectioned plate or not, you imagine you do and think of your plate as being divided into three compartments.

About two thirds of the plate should be full of low-starch vegetables and/or low-glycemic fruits. Because plate and people sizes differ, another way to measure this

ur fruit and vegetable portions to be about the
y ur two fists. This could be a green salad, onions, peppers, chard, kale, asparagus, brussels sprouts, broccoli, spinach, blueberries, blackberries, strawberries, and apples. Eat mostly low-glycemic fruits and vegetables. You will lose weight and control your blood sugar better by focusing on low-glycemic fruit and vegetable choices because fruit contains fiber and natural sugars that won't elevate your blood sugar as quickly as refined sugars will, while vegetables are more complex and contain less sugar. Thus, consuming low-glycemic fruits and vegetables helps you maintain more stable blood-sugar levels while getting the healthy nutrients your body wants from its carbohydrate sources.

If you want to go into more detail about what effect fruits and vegetables can have on your blood sugar and ability to lose weight, I have a chart on the resources page at HowToLiveUntilYouDie.com that you can download for free. That chart shows you how quickly each fruit and vegetable elevates your blood sugar. If you're trying to lose weight or control your blood sugar, this chart will help you identify the best fruits and vegetables for you.

About one third of the plate should be filled with proteins and healthy fats. This includes foods such as nuts and oils, avocados, olives, shrimp, fish, chicken, eggs, and beef. Most people will want to consume about four to six ounces of protein, but to keep it simple and not require you to carry a scale wherever you go, just picture the palm of your hand without the fingers in terms of length, width, and thickness for protein sources and let that be your general measuring device for the proper amount of protein.

Remember, balance is the key. By having each meal include roughly two fists of low-starch vegetables and/or low-glycemic fruits plus a palm-sized portion of protein and healthy fats, you'll make sure each of your meals is more balanced and healthy.

Step 3: Eat three balanced meals.

One of the biggest problems people have is that they don't eat at the right times. Too many people skip breakfast. That's a big mistake. You just fasted for hours—ideally for eight hours of sleep.

When you wake up, your body needs food. It needs a protein-rich breakfast. Many people eat cereal or sugar-rich breakfast options. You need to eat a healthy, protein-rich breakfast and skip the unhealthy alternatives.

If you skip breakfast and your first meal is lunch, you may have gone twelve hours or more before eating. That's not good. That slows your metabolism down.

If you want to control your energy, blood sugar, or weight, you need to eat scheduled meals. It doesn't have to be exact times, but get your breakfast, then 4–5 hours later you need to eat a protein-rich lunch, and 4–5 hours later, you need to eat a healthy dinner. For dinner, you can dial back on the protein if you'd like because protein can be more difficult to digest, leading to interrupted sleep.

If you go more than that long between meals, you need to grab a healthy snack between meals. If you don't, your blood sugar will drop and you'll get irritated and weak, you'll feel the afternoon slump (especially if you eat an imbalanced high-carbohydrate breakfast and high-carbo-hydrate lunch), and your blood sugar will bottom out. You can find more information on healthy snacking in step four.

Step 4: Eat healthy snacks in between meals.

There are a lot of snacks on the market that are hard to resist. Even I want some of them, but most of them are loaded with some or all of the Big Seven Toxins. One of the worst offenders might be one of the most popular one on the market.

I'm talking about cheese-flavored tortilla chips. The next time you're in the snack aisle, compare the label of your favorite flavored tortilla chips to the list of Big Seven Toxins and you'll likely find that you're about to eat a big bag of most or all of them.

Even cereal or protein bars are full of the Big Seven Toxins. Along with breakfast foods, snack foods are big offenders of the Big Seven. Read the labels.

We have so many healthy choices out there that there's no need to eat unhealthy snacks to have a convenient, great-tasting snack. The easiest way to do it is to get a little bit of knowledge up front so you don't have to spend hours of time planning and reading every time you get to the grocery store.

No food tastes as good as it feels to enjoy a more active life doing activities you enjoy.

Finding a few protein bars that you know are clean choices will make it nice and simple to have a cupboard and refrigerator full of healthy snack options. Stock up on nuts, fruit, dark chocolate, real peanut butter (with only peanuts and maybe salt as ingredients), fruit, and vegetables. Any combination of those will be a great start for a simple, healthy snack that tastes great.

Step 5: Start feeling better than ever.

By avoiding the Big Seven Toxins and choosing to eat clean, healthy food, you will begin to look and feel better than ever. Although cutting out processed and fast foods that are full of toxins and proven to lead to obesity and poor health is great, you'll soon realize no food tastes as good as it feels to have energy when you get out of bed in the morning. It's true. No food tastes as good as it feels to enjoy a more active life doing activities you enjoy. No food tastes as good as it feels to get a better health report at ir doctor's office. No food tastes as good as it feels to fit into some favorite old clothes or some new ones. No food tastes as good as it feels to enjoy living a longer, healthier life, and being with your loved ones longer.

Eating healthfully is not just about extending your life, but extending the quality of those years, too. If you want to improve the quantity and quality of life make the right choices. Choose to eat healthier foods. Choose cleaner eating. You'll be happy you did.

Bonus Step:
Consider getting a genetic assessment.

If you want to get more specific with your nutrition, you can obtain a mail-in genetic analysis that will tell you what your specific nutritional needs are based upon your unique DNA. Although this comes with an out-of-pocket cost, it is much more affordable than ever and can give you a detailed analysis that tells you what your body's nutritional needs are, which can help you choose the best foods for your body and help you identify what supplements you may need to take. Many of the tests even come with customized exercise information for your genetic profile as well, which can help you choose the best foods for your body and help you identify what supplements you may need to take.

If you want to learn more about DNA testing, visit HowToLiveUntilYouDie.com.

OPTIMAL LIVING ACTION

1. Commit to incorporating a simple, clean-plan into your life.

2. Avoid fast food for the next 48 hours.

3. Download the glycemic index on the resources page at HowToLiveUntilYouDie.com. Take note of the lower-glycemic fruits and vegetables that you enjoy. Start building a grocery list that includes those.

4. Plan your lunch and dinner mentally ahead of time, even if that just involves spending a few minutes identifying restaurants that have clean options for your lunch break.

CHAPTER 2
EXERCISE

Why You Hate It,
and How to Love It

*"Movement is a medicine for creating change
in a person's physical, emotional,
and mental states."*

– Carol Welch

I F YOU STRUGGLE TO maintain a regular exercise routine, or don't even know how to start, this chapter is for you. In this chapter, I will show you exactly why you and millions of others struggle to exercise regularly, and give you five principles to help you start an exercise program that will work for your body and your lifestyle without having to spend thousands of dollars in gym memberships, workout videos, or personal trainers.

When it comes to feeling good and improving your health, exercise is another area where simple is better. You can't turn on the TV or open a magazine without some guru trying to sell you the next secret exercise program or magic bullet to six-pack abs. With all that information and all those "secrets," you would think that every one of us would be physically fit, yet we all know that is not the case.

I'm here to tell you that all that information is, more often than not, keeping you from reaching your exercise goals instead of pushing you toward them. Exercise has become something people dread. It's seen as complicated, discouraging, painful. It has developed a negative connotation and is even seen as a "dirty word" in the medical area, where professionals have been discouraged from even using the word "exercise." Instead, they are encouraged to use the term "physical activity."

The truth is, exercise is not a dirty word. Exercise can become an incredibly positive and powerful part of your life. All you need to do is apply the five simple principles I give you in this chapter. First let's discuss the problem with most exercise programs.

Most exercise programs have a big problem.

The problem with most exercise programs is not that they don't work. The problem is that they only work when you work. There is no magic pill. There is no shortcut. There is no best exercise program. But there is a best exercise program for you.

I can tell you right now which exercise program is right for you. It's the one that you actually do, over and over again. It's the one you stick with for a long time.

It doesn't matter if the program involves riding a unicycle, juggling watermelons, or training for a triathlon; the most effective program for you is the one that gets you off the couch and moving.

The complicated or extreme exercise programs that you've been pitched by gurus, or their salespeople, often don't work because they are so challenging that you dread doing them. That level of difficulty becomes an excuse for not doing it and you end up doing nothing. In fact, even the idea of doing those extreme exercise programs can add stress to your life and push you further away from exercise and good health.

You can find time to exercise. Here's how.

The idea that you need to join a gym to exercise also keeps people from getting in better shape. Just the thought of sitting through a sales pitch, submitting to a credit check, signing a five-page, four-point font, three-year contract, buying workout clothes, driving to the gym every day, figuring out all the machines, getting pressured to hire a trainer, trying to hide out of the way of the mirrors in a group exercise class, showering at the gym, and so much more, is enough to keep most people dejected and sitting on the couch.

The good news is that I have a solution to all the exercise myths you've been told your entire life. I have a solution that does not require you to install a rock wall on the side of your house or buy an elliptical machine for your basement. There's no sales pitch, no grunting bodybuilders, no three-year contracts, and no one-size-fits-all DVD sets.

Find an exercise program that's built for you.

It's important that any exercise program works with you as an individual and is within your current health limitations. In fact, I'm going to show you how you can even get a workout program designed for your specific DNA. It's definitely important that you consult your doctor or other health-care professional before beginning any exercise routine, but "because a lawyer requires me to say that" is not the reason I'm telling you that. The reason to consult your physician is because exercise is only helpful if the particular program will improve what you need improvement with, while at the same time match your interests and fitness levels so that you can—and actually will—stick with it and gain momentum over time.

The truth is, exercise is not a dirty word.

No matter how many times you've fallen victim to infomercials or extreme exercise fads, then waited six months before another fad got you moving for a few weeks, I can help you get started. I'm not going to prescribe a one-size-fits-all exercise program.

Instead, I'm going to focus on giving you information and simple steps to help you fit exercise into your lifestyle, no matter how long it has been since you last exercised or how little free time you have during the day. This information will help you work with your doctor or other health-care provider to identify activities that will work for you.

Yes, I think you should consult your doctor or other healthcare professional, but it's not just because of legal concerns. I want you to consult your doctor or other healthcare professional after reading this information to make sure you start a program that fits your current health status and actually helps you get results, because there is no plan that works for everyone.

With this information, you'll have all the tools to help you and your doctor or other healthcare provider design a simple plan for exercise to become a part of your lifestyle without trying to force you to install a heavy bag in your basement or spend hours at the gym.

Exercise is about far more than pushups, bench presses, running, or step aerobics, and the benefits of exercise extend far beyond better bathing-suit bodies and smaller pants.

You'll finish this chapter with simple exercise principles that you can begin to implement today so you never get tempted by the latest $99.00, 30day, 25minute, or 7minute supposed "cures" to your exercise woes that have made exercise one of the most misunderstood principles for achieving optimal living.

Exercise is about far more than pushups, bench presses, running, or step aerobics, and the benefits of exercise extend far beyond better bathing-suit bodies and smaller pants. In fact, six packs and smaller clothes are two of the least important benefits of exercise.

Simple may be your only option.

In 2012, my father was diagnosed with chronic lymphocytic leukemia, or CLL, one of two types of lymphocytic leukemia. This cancer debilitates patients and eventually leads to death. People can live for years with CLL before they pass away, although those years are pretty painful. Treatments for CLL are costly and aggressive, with some costing up to $30,000 per treatment, and it requires many treatments.

He immediately began treatments recommended by the doctors. The treatment made him extremely sick. He couldn't function at all, physically, and was nearly broken emotionally, until one Sunday in church, when he found hope in a man whose brother had CLL and was dealing with it very well. Severely debilitated and desperate for relief, my father asked for an introduction, which was arranged.

The man shared several techniques for easing his discomfort and living well with CLL, including adjusting his diet, sleeping with a heated blanket, and other treatments designed to relieve pain on a temporary basis. In addition, the man said getting regular exercise had been nothing short of miraculous for him regarding achieving more permanent pain relief and lifestyle enhancement.

With the level of pain my dad was feeling, telling him to get "regular exercise" sounded as ludicrous as suggesting he jump behind the control panel of a fighter jet. He was in so much pain, so broken, that "regular exercise" was just not going to happen. Even before the CLL diagnosis, he suffered from chronic back pain and diabetes and had been taking medication to manage those conditions. On top of that, he was slowly deteriorating from the CLL and could hardly find the strength to brush his teeth.

After implementing the heated blanket, diet, and other suggestions the man shared with him, there was only one more suggestion remaining: exercise. By that point, the other lifestyle changes had helped him go from practically bedridden to being able to walk very short distances, but he was still in severe pain and discomfort.

> # The only thing you need to do is to move more today than you did yesterday and move tomorrow more than you do today.

For years, his doctors had tried to get him to exercise to help him combat his diabetes, gain strength, and decrease the chronic pain he had been experiencing, but he never did. Ironically, when he was almost completely debilitated by the CLL and the treatments he had been taking, he finally decided it was time to try some exercise. It's strange to me how God works sometimes. Previously, when back pain and sugar levels were his biggest health concerns, he avoided exercise even though numerous experts said it could help him. After CLL ripped him of almost all of his strength, however, to the point that getting out of bed was a chore, he decided it was time to exercise.

What changed? A few things.

First, he was in so much pain and had tried everything else to get comfortable, that exercise became his only hope.

Second, he had been told to exercise so many times that the repetition finally reached his head and his heart.

And third, when complicated exercise programs were no longer an option and the extent of his ability to "exercise" was to take as many steps as he could, all the noise spread by the "fad" fitness community went away. He was left with only one option for exercise: walking. He didn't have to worry about extreme classes, running, stairs, weight lifting, or any one-size-fits-all DVD set. He would just try to take one more step that day than he did the day before.

Exercise, in that context, became simple. Anything more than walking was not an option.

The first day, he walked until he couldn't walk any more, which wasn't very far. The next day, he walked again. Again, he didn't go very far. But by keeping it simple and focusing on getting up and doing what he could—and would—do on a regular basis, he walked farther and farther. After walking became routine, he added doing chores around the house and clearing land by hand, leaving his tractor behind, using chainsaws and swing blades to clean the land manually. In a short time, he went from barely able to get out of bed to walking three to four miles each day, clearing land by hand, and experiencing benefits far beyond that incredible pain relief it ultimately did create in managing his CLL.

At his low point, he was depressed, frequently talking about death and even calling me out of the blue to tell me his wishes for after he passed. As he gained strength, he began living life again. He began enjoying hobbies like singing and playing guitar again. He became much calmer. And, of course, his pain lowered and his overall health improved. He felt good about himself for the first time in a long time.

My father's exercise story is just one illustration of why incorporating a simple exercise program into your life is helpful to achieving an optimal life. There's no need to over complicate things or jump from fad to fad. The only thing you need to do is to move more today than you did yesterday and move tomorrow more than you do today.

His story is also a good illustration that the benefits of regular exercise go beyond bathing suits and pants sizes. In fact, the American Psychological Association, or APA, has shared several studies that found that in addition to improving overall fitness, body mass index, cardiovascular health, and muscular health, exercise and physical activity can "relieve stress, reduce depression, and improve cognitive function."

Indeed, in a 2013 survey by Harris Interactive, Inc., on behalf of the APA, many respondents acknowledged experiencing positive benefits like feeling good about themselves, elevated moods, and less stress, from exercise. Remarkably, however, survey participants still didn't make the time to exercise every day, with more than one third reporting they exercise either not at all or less than once a week.

A simple walk saved my life, too.

I've experienced each of these effects in my life, too. In 2008, I was in the midst of negotiating the sale of my pharmacies for a significant price. I was excited for what we had built for my family and me, and looking forward to the next chapter in my life. Suddenly, however, the economy turned south and the deal fell through. At the same time, we lost a huge government contract, which was the lifeblood of one of my stores.

Within weeks, we went from having strong cash flow, vision into the future, and a large payday from the sale, to barely holding on, struggling to save the business. I held on as long as I could, trying everything I could think of to keep it going, but by December 31, 2009, it was too much and I locked the doors for the last time.

I lost almost everything I had built in my life. It was the end of my dream. I worked for ten years to build and grow a business that I dreamed would provide for the community and my family for years to come. With one turn of the key, the dream was over. We were bankrupt.

I couldn't help but feel the gravity of the situation on my shoulders. The weight of the debt, the guilt, the shame, the stress, and the pain was crushing. What could I have done differently? What could I do next? I had no idea. My confidence was shot.

Over the next weeks and months, I cried more times than I could count; the weight of my emotions was too much to handle. I felt so guilty thinking about all the pain and stress I'd placed on my family.

I started making bad food choices, exercising less, and gaining weight. I was struggling inside and out.

Exercise helped me relieve pain and shame.

I was a mess during that time. I was in deep emotional pain. I was ashamed. I didn't know what to do. One day I decided to take a walk to talk with God, to cry out to God for help and direction without my family hearing.

That first walk led to many more. Whenever I felt my emotions getting the best of me, I'd excuse myself and go for a walk, talk to God, cry, meditate, talk, think, reflect, and pray for direction. I wasn't looking for physical activity or exercise at the time, just some alone time with God. Regardless of my reasons, I began experiencing extraordinary physical and emotional benefits from those walks. The quiet gave me time to process my emotions. The movement calmed my nerves and I could feel my energy rising and my stress falling. I returned from every walk energized and feeling emotionally stronger.

The more I walked, the more areas of my life it affected, too. As my stress levels dropped and my energy increased, I began making healthier food choices and added other exercise to my schedule. The walks became a catalyst for peace and positive momentum in my personal and professional life. They helped me regain my confidence and push me forward to rebuild and refocus.

Working movement into your day will help you build momentum for your future.

Before I started taking walks, I was so stressed that the idea of starting a formal workout program would have sent me straight to the couch. I didn't have the energy or brainpower to take on that challenge, but because I kept it simple, quietly walking to talk with God and get my body moving, I found peace and began building momentum that I'm still building upon today.

The same can be true for you. Exercise is a critical pillar to living an optimal life. Whether you're struggling move a few feet like my dad was, feeling emotionally broken like I was in 2009–2010, or sitting in traffic all morning just to sit at a desk all day and then sit in more traffic on the way home, arriving home mentally drained from a stressful day, working movement into your day will help you build momentum for your future.

Keeping it simple is key, so forget about all those DVDs or extreme bodybuilding routines, and just start moving more. To help you get started, here are six principles of healthy exercise that you can use to work a simple, custom exercise program into your life. Call your doctor, or reach out to me directly, if you want help working any of these principles into your life, and visit the resources page at HowToLiveUntilYouDie.com for more information and direction. We can help you get started.

1. Keep it simple.

You know by now that simpler is better for the long term. Start by moving more today than you did yesterday. Get off the couch and go for a walk around the block. Mow the lawn with a push mower instead of a tractor.

2. Be consistent and compete only against yourself.

Don't overdo it. Work on consistency and improvement. Work on doing more tomorrow than today. Don't concern yourself with your neighbor's crazy exercise routine. Challenge yourself and compete only against yourself. Your body will thank you.

3. Focus on moving more during your daily routine.

Americans are living a more sedentary lifestyle than ever before. Many of our jobs confine us to a desk and more days than not we're so tired and stressed when we get home, that we go straight to the couch, shovel uninspiring convenience food in our mouths, and head to bed to watch the latest reality show. Our bodies are crying out for activity and we have to answer the call.

Research shows that it is best to be active at least every ninety minutes and that simple activity throughout the day increases blood flow, enhances concentration, and boosts energy levels. By setting an alarm on your phone to go off every sixty to ninety minutes to remind you to get up and move for a few minutes, you can experience some of these benefits for yourself and move toward a less sedentary lifestyle. Keep it simple, but keep moving.

To help you design something that would work for you, here's an example of what a Work Day Movement Program might look like. If you want to see me demonstrate these exercises, go to the resources page at HowToLiveUntilYouDie.com:

7:45 – Arrive at work fifteen minutes early, if you can, after a healthy breakfast. Take a fifteen-minute walk before your day starts. This will help you to get some steps in and help you feel great and ready for a productive day!

9:30 – Time for first break. Jump up and push your chair under your desk and do two or three sets of Air Squats. Place your feet shoulder-width apart and your arms stretched out in front of you. Bend your knees while keeping your back straight and your head up. Do fifteen in a row and take a one-minute rest between sets. If you can't do squats at work because of dress codes or shared space, a ten-minute walk will do just fine. The point is to get up and get moving for ten minutes.

9:40 – Back to work, feeling good!

11:10 – Lunch may be coming soon, but before you go eat, do two or three sets of Desk Dips. Place your chair to the side and face away from your desk. With the desk to your back, put your palms on the desk with your knees slightly bent in front of you. Dip down until your elbows form ninety-degree angles and then push yourself back up. Do ten in a row and take a one-minute rest between sets. For added difficulty, place your feet in your chair. (Be extra careful with that one.) Just like with the morning movements, if you can't do desk dips at work, take another walk during this time.

12:30 – Back from lunch and back to the grind!

2:00 – This next exercise is a core, hamstring, and leg exercise that you don't have to leave your chair for, but you will need to turn it around to face away from the desk. It's the Wooden Leg! Place your hands on the chair by your sides, keeping your back straight and one foot flat on the floor. Raise the other foot straight in front of you. Hold it there for five seconds, and then raise it as high as you can for five seconds. Exercise each leg ten times. Again, don't worry if you can't exercise at your desk. Just make sure to get up and get moving for ten minutes.

2:10 – On the home stretch!

3:40 – Final exercise for the day is a twist on an oldie but goodie: Desk Push-Ups. Place your chair to the side and place your hands on the desk while facing it. Keep your back and legs straight and drop your body until your elbows are at ninety degrees and then push yourself up. Perform two or three sets of ten, taking a one-minute break in between sets. For added difficulty, drop down on the floor for traditional pushups. If you need to substitute walking again, that's just fine. With four walking sessions, you're building up your steps! If you hit 10,000 steps per day, your body can shed one to two pounds per week, so if you aren't walking and can add 10,000 steps per day, you can not only start feeling better, but you can get help losing weight, too! Most smartphones have built-in step counters, too, so you can just leave your phone in your pocket and walk away.

3:50 – Only one hour left between you and the door! Finish strong with the extra energy you've given yourself from staying active!

There are plenty of other ways to stay active at work as well. Replacing your chair with an exercise ball increases core strength and improves posture. Another option that is becoming increasingly common is using a standup desk. I even have a friend who goes to another floor to use the restroom, and takes the stairs up and down to get there. It only takes a few extra seconds, too.

Another great way to minimize the negative effects of sitting in a chair all day is to alternate between standing and sitting at your desk. If you're fortunate enough to have a standing desk, or one that can shift between standing and sitting, that's ideal. If not, don't worry. Designate tasks that you do frequently and don't require you to be sitting in your chair as "standing tasks." This might include conference calls, reading reports, checking the mail, or listening to voicemail. If that's not practical for your job, try finding a way to shift between standing and sitting, perhaps standing fifteen minutes every hour.

4. Learn your body and what works best for you.

Yes, this means talking to your doctor or other healthcare provider to make sure your exercise program is not harmful to your specific needs. Your healthcare provider knows what health issues you are dealing with and can help you choose movement that will be beneficial to you. If your doctor or other health-care provider can't or won't talk with you about what specific exercise would work for you, ask for a referral to someone who can assess your specific health and exercise needs. Some health-care providers prefer not to instruct on specific exercise programs. Don't let one health-care provider's inability or refusal to help you keep you from getting that help from someone else.

Be realistic and start slow. Listen to your body as you begin your program. Monitor how consistent you are. If you find yourself skipping workouts, it might be time to change, because something about that routine doesn't work for you. Finally, if you want to find an exercise program that is built for your unique makeup, becoming your own guru may be just the thing you need to start achieving meaningful results.

5. Become your own guru.

We live in a world where science and technology are advancing rapidly. This gives us access to more and better information at a fraction of the cost of only a few years ago and at much faster speeds than ever before. Take advantage of that to simplify and customize an exercise program that is designed for your body and is within your fitness levels.

Although this suggestion requires an initial out-of-pocket cost, this is my favorite exercise tip because the benefits it can provide can help you become your own exercise guru and avoid fad exercise programs for the rest of your life.

I'm talking about getting a mail-in genetic analysis conducted. I know it sounds complicated. That may have been true years ago. Genetic testing is now simple, affordable, and available to the masses. In fact, it's as easy as buying a kit, swabbing your cheek or spitting in a test tube, and mailing the sample to a lab in a prepaid envelope.

The lab then analyzes your DNA and sends you a detailed analysis along with exercise plans that are personalized to your individual genetic profile. Some labs even provide genetically guided nutrition advice as well. With that report, you and your doctor can supercharge your exercise program based on an analysis of your body, while staying within your current fitness levels.

The results of the genetic testing can help you be more efficient and effective with your exercise program. For example, when I had my DNA analyzed, the results told me that the most effective exercise regime for me is roughly half power exercises and half endurance exercises and gave me lists of exercises that fell into those categories.

A client of mine was surprised to discover that his exercise program was far from ideal for his genetic profile. He had been spending 90% of his exercise time on endurance exercises and only 10% on power exercises. His DNA test told him he should be doing the opposite, 90% power to 10% endurance.

As of this writing, you can get genetic testing with a custom-designed diet and exercise program for less than one of those one-size-fits-all, ninety-day extreme home workout programs plus the equipment you'd need for those programs.

If you want to learn more about DNA testing, visit HowToLiveUntilYouDie.com.

6. Get help.

No matter how dedicated you are or how simple your plan is, exercise is harder if you're doing it alone. Whether it's getting out of your warm bed in the cold winter months, staying consistent during a busy season, or giving an extra effort during your exercise sessions, it's harder when the only person pushing you is yourself. Because of that, I highly recommend that you get help. This could be in the form of a friend or relative who exercises with you, a personal or group trainer at your local fitness center, a private trainer, or an online or in-person accountability group.

I did this myself a few months ago, hiring an incredible fitness trainer named Jeff McMahon to help me. Jeff and I meet virtually over Skype. He helps me stay on track with my fitness and pushes me to do more than I would do on my own. He's single-handedly helped me take my fitness to a higher level than I ever could on my own.

If you can afford to hire someone who is a trained fitness professional like Jeff, I highly recommend it. By investing your own money into the advice and accountability, it tends to add an additional layer of commitment as well. If a professional trainer is not in your budget, consider a workout partner, group walks, exercise or yoga classes, or some other way to stay accountable and motivated.

OPTIMAL LIVING ACTION STEPS

1. Commit to working more movement into your life. Take a daily walk. Take movement breaks at work. Do pushups every morning. The details don't matter, but getting started does. Write down one thing you are going to do, starting today, to begin: _____ _____.

2. Review two genetic-testing options and consider getting your personal exercise suggestions completed. If you need help finding some, head on over to the resources page at HowToLiveUntilYouDie.com for a few suggestions.

3. Put those DVDs and extreme programs in a box and forget about them. Sell them if you want, or throw them away. Cancel any memberships you haven't used in months where you don't have a contractual commitment, or at least freeze your membership. You may build up to those or choose to go back as you build momentum, but for now, those DVDs and gym memberships are a drain on

your mind and your money, reminders of the hope you placed in the system (or salespeople) who told you they would be your solution.

4. Reach out to your doctor with any questions or to help you design a simple exercise program that you can—and will—do. I am here for you, too.

Just go to HowToLiveUntilYouDie.com and you can schedule a time to talk with me or sign up to receive daily encouragement from me and I'll send you an email every day with simple exercise tips and encouragement to get help you get motivated, get moving, and remain accountable.

WATER

The Simple Solution to Many Mental and Physical Ailments

"Drinking water is like washing out your insides. The water will cleanse the system, fill you up, decrease your caloric load and improve the function of all your tissues."

– Kevin R. Stone

IF YOU ASK MOST people how much water they're supposed to drink in a day, the most common answer will be "eight glasses." Yet if you ask the followup question about how much they actually drink in a day, you'll likely hear a number that's much less than that.

I know. As a pharmacist, I encounter people every day with all kinds of health problems, who come to me seeking counsel on natural solutions to their ailments, so they don't have to take prescription medications. One of the first questions I ask them is how much water they're drinking in a day. I have asked thousands of people this question, only to hear "not nearly enough," over and over again.

When pressed further, the reasons given for not drinking enough water are the same:

- It tastes too plain.
- It's too boring.
- My tap water tastes bad.
- If I drink all that water, I'll spend half the day in the bathroom.
- I refuse to pay for water.
- I love (or need) my morning coffee or tea.
- I need a sports drink for energy and during sports.
- I need the caffeine jolt from my sodas.
- I need to have my energy drinks or coffee or tea, and if I add enough water to that, I would be drinking all day.

- I am drinking diet sodas, so it's not like I'm getting a lot of sugar.
- I'm getting hydrated from my coffee, tea, soda, or sports drinks.

I certainly understand those responses and have felt that way about some of them in the past, but as I looked deeper into both water and the alternative drinks, I've come to realize that much of the negative sentiments toward water are unfounded and many of the objections are the result of marketing rather than data. At the same time, I have found much of the positive information about other drinks, especially sports drinks, to be equally unfounded.

This misinformation is causing people to drink far too little water and far too many drinks that are loaded with toxic dyes, artificial flavors and other chemicals that can be so harmful and far outweigh any hydration or jolt of energy you get from drinking those neon-colored elixirs, sodas, or melted ice cream with a shot of espresso that some companies pass off as coffee.

This dilemma is especially challenging for parents of children who are exposed to misinformation about sports drinks. For example, I recently worked with a mother of a ten-year-old boy who was a great athlete, but was experiencing severe weakness and headaches. They couldn't figure out what the problem was until I advised them to switch from the sports drinks he was drinking to pure water. Shortly after switching, the weakness went away and the headaches stopped. After some more research, we came to find out that one of the dyes in the sports drinks was causing the weakness and headaches and switching to water kept him feeling good and well hydrated.

Another client and friend of mine, Aaron Walker, was suffering from severe back pain. He tried everything he could think of to resolve his pain, from stretching, to strengthening, to therapy. Nothing worked. As part of an overall health plan, Aaron and I evaluated where he was with each of the seven N.E.W.S.S.S.S. key areas of his life. He was strong in many of the areas, however his water intake was severely lacking, so one of the first things he did was start drinking more water. It turned out water intake was the final piece of the puzzle for Aaron. Within weeks, the back pain that had plagued him for years disappeared. Aaron didn't have a back problem. He had a water problem. He was dehydrated.

Water is so important that no matter what ailment the person is asking about, one of the first questions I ask is how much water they're drinking a day. The most common answer I receive in response to that is "not nearly enough," and they're telling the truth. Sadly, that's the truth for most people today.

I believe the vast majority of people walking around the earth today have a form of mild dehydration because too many people are drinking coffees, sodas, and sports drinks, and not enough people are consuming enough

Chapter 3: Water

water, contributing to hundreds of thousands of deaths every year.

Because our bodies are the temple of the Holy Spirit, it is our duty to make sure we are treating it as such. Over the past two-plus decades, I have both studied and witnessed the effect of replacing chemical-based elixirs marketed as enhanced water, infused water, or sports drinks—in addition to sodas and diet sodas—with water. I've seen energy levels rise, pain disappear, strength and stamina increase, and more after simple switches from sugary or chemical-filled drinks to water. Getting enough water is a critically important part of a balanced plan to be more happy, healthy, and whole.

Why do we need water?

We can't live without water. Our bodies consist primarily of water. We're made out of water and dirt, gas and minerals, because that's what water is: liquified gas made out of hydrogen and oxygen. We need water to survive. It needs to be replenished. We even need water for our bodies to make more blood.

Although a lot of these facts have been widely discussed for decades, the attention paid to dehydration and water consumption became unavoidable in the medical community after a groundbreaking 1995 book, *Your Body's Many Cries for Water: You're Not Sick, You're Thirsty; Don't Treat Thirst with Medication*, by Dr. Fereydoon

49

Batmanghelidj was published. It made several alarming observations about the effect of dehydration, including that dehydration leads to stress, chronic pains, and many painful degenerative diseases, and that over 75% of Americans are chronically dehydrated. According to Dr. Batmanghelidj, over one third of Americans are so dehydrated that their thirst mechanisms are weakened to the point that thirst is often mistaken with hunger, and even mild dehydration can slow your metabolism by 3%. This suggests that water can be an important part of any plan to burn fat, lose weight, and speed up your metabolism.

The effects of dehydration are more immediate than slower metabolisms or weight gain, too, Dr. Batmanghelidj warned, noting that lack of water is the number-one trigger of daytime fatigue and a mere 2% drop in body water can reduce short-term memory, inhibit basic mental functions like performing basic math equations, and cause difficulty in focusing on a computer screen or printed page. This suggests that there are kids who are having trouble with school work who might just be dehydrated.

On the other hand, Dr. Batmanghelidj contended, water intake has been observed to ease back and joint pain, shut down midnight hunger pangs, and even reduce certain cancer risks by 45–79%. In cases of the common cold or flu, increasing your water intake can reduce the number of sick days by two to three days, Dr. Batmanghelidj advised. In other words, water can be medicinal, too.

Is water really a solution?

Let's dig deeper into the science. *Your Body's Many Cries for Water* has been a matter of heated debate, as it called a lot of traditional thought into doubt, arguing that water might be the answer to many mental and physical ailments. In the decades since it was released, the medical and scientific community conducted several studies about the effect of water and dehydration on health.

Although published studies don't evaluate every claim made by Dr. Batmanghelidj, several reputable studies confirmed substantial negative mental and physical health consequences of dehydration as well as the specific importance of drinking enough water.

For example, in its January 15, 2004 edition, the *Journal of Clinical Oncology* published a response to an article on cancer prevention submitted by Yair Bar David, Benjamin Gesundheit, Jacob Urkin, and Joseph Kapelushnik, Child Health Center and Pediatric Hematology and Oncology, Soroka Medical Center, Beer Sheva, Israel. The reply noted that, while the article on cancer prevention listed several factors of cancer prevention, it failed to address the proven role of fluid intake and, specifically, water.[9]

The article also referenced several studies that found statistically significant correlations between water and fluid intake and cancer risk, including reducing risks of bladder cancer, rectal cancer, colorectal cancer, colon cancer, and breast cancer.[10]

y to water, studies cited included conclu-
Vater intake alone was significantly associ-
luced risk of colon cancer" for both men and
"water drinking appeared strongly inversely
and significantly associated with breast cancer risk."[11]

Additionally, in 2012, two studies from the University of Connecticut's Human Performance Laboratory linked mild dehydration with altered mood, lower energy levels, and lessened abilities to think clearly.[12]

Finally, a peer-reviewed manuscript published on behalf of the International Life Sciences Institute went further. It explored the status of all research on water intake and health, looking to clear up questions about water and health and "encourage more dialogue on this important topic."[13]

After its comprehensive review, the authors declare with no hesitation that "The effects of water on daily performance and short and long-term health are quite clear" and that water is "undoubtedly the most important nutrient and the only one whose absence will be lethal within days."[14]

Collectively, these analyses along with dozens if not hundreds of others have concluded hydration and water intake are critical to long-term health and can even have medicinal effects. There can be no doubt anymore that water is essential. The only question that remains is how to ensure that you get as many of the benefits as possible, in a way that keeps it simple and works with your budget and lifestyle.

Other drinks aren't good enough.

One of the loudest objections to drinking water in place of other drinks like sodas, vitamin-infused water, or sports drinks is that those drinks either offer specialized tastes or vitamins and minerals (such as the electrolytes sodium, potassium, chloride, calcium, magnesium, bicarbonate, phosphate, and sulfate), which our bodies need to function properly.

When it comes to sodas, the conclusion is obvious. Although you will get somewhat hydrated by drinking sodas, sodas offer few if any vitamins or minerals, and are loaded with chemicals such as artificial colors, sweeteners, and flavors.

When it comes to vitamin-infused water and sports drinks, although I agree that our bodies need vitamins, minerals, and electrolytes, I disagree with the suggestion that the only way for you to get them is to drink infused water or sports drinks instead of water.

In fact, if you attend to all seven key areas of life that the N.E.W.S.S.S.S. acronym walks you through for optimal health, you will be able to get all the vitamins, minerals, and electrolytes your body needs from natural sources, such as healthy food and clean supplements, which I'll talk about in Chapter 5.

You can also add electrolytes to a bottle of spring water yourself by adding a little Himalayan salt, which provides sodium and chloride as well as small amounts of other electrolytes, such as potassium and magnesium. If you aren't able to get Himalayan salt, sea salt is the next best option, although the levels of potassium and magnesium in sea salt are much lower than in Himalayan salt. This helps you avoid sugary or chemical-filled drinks while still getting the minerals and electrolytes your body needs. All you have to do is just mix it into your water.

Drink the best water.

After decades of analysis, it's now undeniable that drinking water is essential to your health, especially as part of a balanced nutrition and supplement program like this. Water, thus, is the simplest and best drinking choice for your health.

But there are so many options, how do you know what type of water to drink to make sure you're getting the most benefits, and great taste, while keeping it simple and consistent with your lifestyle? Where is the right balance?

It used to be assumed that water is water. Older generations believed that because they drank tap water, everyone should. The truth is that tap water is the worst kind of water to drink because it's often full of chemicals. In fact, even the United States Environmental Protection Agency, or EPA, concedes:

Drinking water can reasonably be expected to contain at least small amounts of some contaminants. As long as those contaminants are at levels no higher than EPA standards, the water is considered safe to drink for healthy people. People with severely weakened immune systems or other specific health conditions, or those concerned about specific contaminants present in local drinking water, may wish to further treat their water at home or purchase high quality bottled water."[15]

In addition, according to a 2013 report in *Scientific American*, "Traces of 18 unregulated chemicals were found in drinking water from more than one-third of U.S. water utilities in a nationwide sampling, according to new, unpublished research by federal scientists."[16] The chemicals included "11 perfluorinated compounds, an herbicide, two solvents, caffeine, an antibacterial compound, a metal, and an antidepressant."[17] Although the effects the chemicals have on humans wasn't known at the time, one of them had been linked to a variety of health problems, including cancer, among people in communities with water contamination.[18]

Because those 18 chemicals were not regulated by the EPA, utilities don't have to meet a limit or even monitor for them. Even though the levels were generally low, a research hydrologist with the U.S. Geological Survey who participated in the study indicated that "there's still the unknown" and pondered whether there were any "long-term consequences of low-level exposure to these chemicals."[19]

Finally, in 2016, additional studies reported that millions of Americans' tap water was full of dangerous chemicals. First, in August 2016, an analysis found that millions of Americans' tap water included unacceptable levels of poly- and perflouroalkyl substances, which pose risks to developmental, immune, metabolic, and endocrine health.[20] Additionally, in September 2016, the Environmental Working Group, an independent advocacy group, released an analysis based upon evidence from water systems throughout the United States that concluded that the tap water of 218 million Americans contained levels of chromium-6, a chemical made famous by Erin Brockovich and the movie *A Civil Action*, which is known to cause cancer, liver damage, reproductive problems, and developmental harm.[21]

If tap water were reliable, I'd be the first person to tell you to drink it. But the fact is it's not, and dangerous chemicals are flowing through the pipes and the taps you would be drinking from if you drank tap water. In fact, hundreds of millions of people are being served tap water full of toxic chemicals. Because of that, I highly recommend avoiding tap water. If you choose to drink tap water, at the very least use a filtration system either on the tap itself, or in a pitcher to filter out the chemicals. Filtration can be effective; however, it can be inconsistent and the lifespan of the filters can weaken its effectiveness over time, making your hazardous chemical consumption a matter of "how much" instead of eliminating it altogether.

On the other end of the spectrum, the most reliable way to ensure you're getting the best tasting and beneficial water is through direct access to a clean well or spring. For most Americans, though, this is either prohibitively expensive or impossible, since digging and maintaining a well can be expensive, and clean springs aren't found on every street corner.

Because of that, I highly recommend drinking high-quality bottled spring or mineralized water. This ensures you get the best tasting, best-for-you source of hydration as reasonably possible without adjusting your lifestyle or breaking the bank. Spring water contains many of the minerals and electrolytes your body needs, tastes clean, and with a squeeze of fresh lemon or lime—or the use of a chemical-free, naturally taste-changing cup like *The Right Cup*, which came to market in 2016,[22]—it can taste even better than the chemical-infused elixirs marketed as sports drinks or enhanced waters. I've found most people who consistently work on all seven N.E.W.S.S.S.S. key areas of life enjoy the taste of spring water, along with its positive contributions to their mental and physical health.

If bottled spring water is not available, bottled purified water is a second-best choice. It's essentially the bottled version of filtered tap water, so it comes with diminished

ity, but it'll do in a pinch. Either way, most bott-
ater has a history of being safe. One caution with
bottled water is that you want to store the bottles in a
cool, dark place. Because the bottles are made of plastic, if
they're stored in the heat or direct sunlight, the chemicals
from the plastic could leach into the water. So if you're
pulling up to a store and see bottled water piled up outside, avoid those and get your water from the shelf inside
or the cooler.

My favorite type of water, and the type I drink most
often, especially when at home, is alkaline ionized water.
I have a machine at home, called a Kangen machine, that
filters and cleanses water while alkalizing and ionizing the
water. Alkaline ionized water has become more popular
as people invest more time and money learning about the
benefits of water and how they can improve their health by
changing both the type and amount of water they drink.

Alkaline ionized water helps counteract acidic things
we put in our bodies, such as some of the Seven Big Toxins, coffee, alcohol, some meat products, and soda. Your
body's acidic or alkalized level is measured on a scale
between zero and fourteen. Anything above 7 is considered alkaline, while anything below 7 is considered acidic.

According to a study published by the *Journal of Environmental and Public Health* in 2011, the ideal pH level is
a slightly alkaline 7.4.[23] Thus, counteracting the frequent
acidic inputs is important.

The same 2011 study found that a diet that focused on higher alkaline levels may have several health benefits including better bone health, reduced muscle wasting, mitigation of some chronic diseases such as hypertension or strokes; it may improve many outcomes from cardiovascular health to memory and cognition, increase intracellular magnesium (which can help activate vitamin D in your body) and perhaps provide added benefit for some chemotherapeutic agents.[24]

In addition, many people have found that alkaline ionized water also tastes even better and smoother than tap, filtered, or spring water. I also find that, unlike other types of water, alkaline ionized water doesn't cause the same bloated feeling that often results from drinking water.

If you're interested in learning more about alkalized ionized water, you can find more information about what I use and why on the resources page at HowToLiveUntilYouDie.com.

The bottom line is, we need to be drinking more water and there's no adequate replacement for pure spring water to get you the great benefits of water without breaking your bank account or disrupting your lifestyle. Your health depends on it.

Work water into your lifestyle.

Now that we know there is no substitute for good spring water for health purposes, let's talk more about ng it into your lifestyle. Water is no different than

ition, exercise, or the rest of the N.E.W.S.S.S.S. key

areas of life in that it does you no good unless the program is simple enough to fit your lifestyle. With water, this means to make sure you get the right amount of water at the right times of the day. Fortunately, these few simple guidelines can help you do just that.

There are two rules of thumb when trying to figure out how much water to drink a day. The first rule of thumb is to drink half an ounce of water for every pound you weigh, spread out throughout the day. So if you're 192 pounds, you should aim for 96 ounces of water, or approximately six standard-sized bottles of spring water per day. The second rule of thumb is to drink enough water that your urine is a pale straw color. One sign that you're not drinking enough water or that you're drinking too much of something else—especially something with an artificial dye—is that your urine is dark yellow, or another color. If your urine isn't pale, you're drinking too much of something else, or at least not drinking enough water. If, on the other hand, your urine has no color or is transparent, you may be drinking too much water and may need to cut back some.[25]

The other consideration for working water into your lifestyle is to drink it at the right times that support proper hydration and don't disrupt your lifestyle. These five simple guidelines will help you do exactly that.

First, it's important to get your day started out with proper hydration in mind. Keep one or two cups of pure water next to your bed and drink it first thing in the morning. You've just gone hours without any water, so starting your day by replenishing the water your body used during sleep is critical. It's perfectly fine to have a little coffee or tea in the morning as well, especially if you aren't adding unhealthy chemicals or sugars to it, but don't let that substitute for one or two cups of water to kickstart your daily hydration.

Second, carry a small jug or bottle of water with you and sip from it throughout the day, even before you get thirsty. Thirst is our body's way of telling us it needs water, so if you wait to drink until you feel thirsty, you may already be partially dehydrated.

Third, drink one glass of water before you eat. This helps get the gastric juices flowing in your stomach and improves digestion. You can sip water during your meal, too, but drinking a full glass of water about ten to fifteen minutes before you eat you will help your body prepare to digest and can help you feel less hungry, so you eat less as well.

Fourth, know your schedule. If you have a one-hour meeting, avoid drinking water for the hour before and use the restroom before the meeting. Toward the middle or end of the meeting, you can start sipping water again, but getting hydrated early in your day and sipping it throughout allows you to remain hydrated and make sure you minimize any emergency and inconvenient trips to the restroom.

Finally, don't drink too much water after dinner, because although hydration is an important part of your total health plan, ensuring you get the right amount of uninterrupted sleep is another important part of a balanced plan. Instead, drink one cup of water after dinner, then right before bed, use the restroom and sip a few ounces of water with a bit of salt for extra electrolytes. This will give you enough hydration and minerals to serve your body while you rest without disrupting your sleep—the next essential part of living a happy, healthy, and vibrant, feeling good life.

OPTIMAL LIVING ACTION STEPS

1. Commit to incorporating quality bottled spring or filtered water into your lifestyle.

2. Drink one or two cups of pure water every morning when you wake up. If you can, add some lemon juice to it. The lemon will not only taste great, but the lemon juice can also benefit your liver and boost your metabolism.

3. Replace your regular beverage with bottled water when you eat out. If you struggle to do this, limit yourself to one other drink and substitute water for the refills.

CHAPTER 4
SLEEP

How to Fall Asleep, Stay Asleep, and Feel Rested

*"A good laugh and a long sleep
are the best cures in the doctor's book."*

– Irish Proverb

THE IMPORTANCE OF SLEEP has been cited by the world's most successful people at least as far back as Aristotle, who wrote in *On Sleep and Sleeplessness* about the importance of sleep in 350 B.C.,[26] and most everyone can finish Ben Franklin's famous proverb "early to bed, early to rise, makes a man healthy, wealthy, and wise."

Sleep has always been widely considered important, yet many people find themselves giving up precious sleep time in a desperate attempt to be more productive; others are so stressed or depressed that they don't get quality sleep, and still others get inconsistent sleep at best. In fact, in February 2016, the Centers for Disease Control and Prevention released data indicating that over a third of American adults don't get enough sleep.[27]

An estimate shared by *Consumer Reports* indicated that approximately 164 million Americans struggle to get a good night's sleep at least once a week.[28] This statistic is hardly surprising given the many pulls on our time, along with the many stresses, distractions, and pressures these days. At home, our spouses, kids, and extended family are busier than ever. We are also more stressed than ever from family and work obligations. We seem to be working longer and harder than ever before, with about 20% of Americans working at least 60 hours per week[29] only to come home after a long, stressful day at work to sports and activities, kids' homework, house chores, and more.

When we finally lie down to bed, our minds continue to race and worry. It seemingly never ends. At the end of the day, all the pulls, pressures, and interruptions leave us overworked, stressed out, and desperate for rest.

Additionally, according to the National Sleep Foundation, 95% of people use "some kind of computer, video game, or cell phone at least a few nights a week within the hour before bed." Those gadgets and screens suppress melatonin, a hormone your body produces that helps control sleep and wake cycles, keep your brain alert, and even wake you up.[30]

> *"The person who takes medicine*
> *must recover twice,*
> *once from the disease and*
> *once from the medicine."*
> **– William Osler, M.D.**

With all those things stacked against us, it's no wonder so many people don't get enough sleep. I've been there, too. I've spent nights worrying about my wife, kids, pharmacies, and more. I've been stressed. I've been depressed. I can't count how many nights I spent with my mind racing, tossing and turning for hours.

I've also worked with thousands of people just like you who were overworked and stressed, pulled from obligation to obligation and left empty and unable to wind down at the end of the day. I've watched people pick up prescription sleep aids month after month, desperate for just one good night's sleep.

In 2013, the Centers for Disease Control and Prevention released data from a five-year survey that indicated nearly 9 million Americans used prescription sleep aids,[31] many of which have been found to help people get an average of only eight to twenty minutes of extra sleep, often with side effects like next-day drowsiness.[32]

The only solutions that I've seen actually work over the long term, for most people, have the same two qualities as the other N.E.W.S.S.S.S. key areas of life: information and simplicity. Without information about why—and how—to get better and more sleep on a regular basis, it's easy to slip back into trying to "power through" another night, week, or month without getting adequate sleep, thinking short-term sleep deprivation can make you more productive. Similarly, Americans spend approximately $41 billion per year on expensive, awkward, ineffective, or uncomfortable sleep aids and remedies,[33] many of which are often wastes of money.

For most people, the solution to better sleep doesn't lie in another expensive sleep aid or prescription medication. The solution is far simpler than that. Before we get into how you can get more and better sleep, however, it's important to understand why sleep is so important and the consequences of not getting enough quality of sleep.

We were designed to sleep.

We all know that we cannot function from day to day without proper sleep. We can feel the effects of sleep deprivation on our bodies and minds. The less we get and the longer the deprivation lasts, the worse we function and feel. We all know this from a general perspective, yet even I resisted for years, regularly sleeping no more than five hours per day.

No matter how much I learned or how much I knew, I constantly fought back against getting enough sleep, thinking I was an exception to the rule, that my body didn't need it or my mind could withstand it. Not even falling asleep behind the wheel and totaling my car set me straight. I thank God every time I think of that day that He had me surrounded by angels and I was able to walk away unscathed because many people who fall asleep behind the wheel don't make it.

It wasn't until I looked at sleep as a whole, three-part being consisting of body, soul, *and spirit*, that I began to let go of my ill-conceived belief that sleep time didn't matter as much as my time awake. When I saw the many references to Jesus sleeping and the importance of sleep in the Bible, I began to see that sleep was more important than just a way to rest and replenish our bodies. In fact, one of my favorite stories in the Bible, from Mark 4:35–41, starts with Jesus sleeping in the back of a boat when a fierce storm and high waves rattled the boat, threatening to drown all occupants. The disciples were scared and woke Him shouting, "Teacher, don't you care that we're going to drown?" But Jesus woke up, rebuked the wind, and demanded the waves to be still. The waves stopped, a great calm ensued, and the disciples' faith was elevated.

If even Jesus slept, and slept while crossing a lake during a fierce storm with high waves crushing the boat, what does that tell me about the importance of sleep? And when He woke up and turned to the storm and the waves that caused His sleep to be interrupted by the disciples out of fear, what does that tell us to do with the earthly worries or desires that interrupt our own sleep?

Sleep is far more than just rest for the body, I realized. It is how God created us. He created us to sleep for almost one third of our lives. He just as easily could have made us to not need sleep at all, but instead He masterfully made us so that our body needs sleep to function.

The more I examined it, the more I was convinced that we are designed to sleep, the more I let go of the one-dimensional belief that sleep didn't matter, and the more I realized that I, too, needed to tell the Earthly storms that kept me from sleeping to stop. Although this is still a major struggle for me, as operating on four to five hours of sleep has been my way of life, I'm working hard every day to get at least seven quality hours of sleep and tell my storms to stop.

Regarding sleep matters, take a scientific approach.

Sleep is one of the most well-researched topics in the scientific community, with countless studies evaluating the effects of sleep on your mental, emotional, and physical health. The results are clear and consistent and there is no doubt that getting enough quality sleep is essential to living a healthy, vibrant, feeling good life.

For example, according to the National Sleep Foundation, research has shown that "the shorter length of time a person sleeps, the greater their risk of being obese,"[34] which is well established as having significant negative effects on long-term health. Researchers from St. Luke's Roosevelt Hospital Center and Columbia University in New York associate lack of sleep with junk-food cravings.[35]

It doesn't end there, either. Dr. Eric J. Olson from the Mayo Clinic summarized studies that show "people who don't get quality or enough sleep are more likely to get sick after being exposed to a virus, such as the common cold virus" and "also affect how fast you recover if you do get sick."[36]

Other studies found insufficient sleep is associated with significant increases with risky behavior in teenagers, such as considering suicide, smoking cigarettes, drinking alcohol, drinking soda, being physically inactive, feeling sad or hopeless, using marijuana, being sexually active, and getting into physical fights.[37]

Another study found that both total and partial sleep deprivation inhibit cognitive performance, such as attention, working memory, long-term memory, decision-making, attention, and vigilance.[38] Researchers have also found a link between poor sleep and diabetes.[39] On the other hand, adequate sleep keeps you alert and helps your brain function last throughout the day, according to Bronwyn Fryer, who reported in the *Harvard Business Review* that sleep deficit is a "performance killer."[40]

It gets worse. According to the European Society of Cardiology, a study determined that poor sleep is associated with increased risk of heart attack and stroke.[41] A peer-reviewed study published in the scientific journal *Sleep* even associated getting too little—or too much—sleep with premature death, calling too little or too much sleep "significant predictors" of death.[42]

In addition to avoiding mental, emotional, and physical health consequences of too little, too much, or poor-quality sleep, getting the right amount of quality sleep has been associated with greater college academic performance,[43] and even higher income, according to research conducted by Matthew Gibson of the University of California, San Diego, who concluded that after investigating the relationship between sleep and wages and ruling out alternative hypotheses, sleep influenced long-term wages by nearly five percent.[44]

Finally, University of Chicago scientists found that

poor sleep patterns had incredibly negative consequences in men, in particular, significantly lowering testosterone levels, which has been associated with reduced libido, poor reproduction, lower muscle mass, reduced bone density, Type 2 diabetes, and more.[45] What results is what I've termed S.E.L. Deficiency Syndrome, which stands for Sleep, Energy, and Libido Deficiency Syndrome, and which is characterized by men spending most of their days and nights like walking zombies with little energy, libido, or sleep.

The studies are consistent and clear. Getting the right amount and quality of sleep is essential for health and productivity. Too little sleep, too much sleep, or poor sleep can hurt you in the short and long-term,[46] and even kill you. On the other hand, getting the right amount of quality sleep can make you healthier, happier, and more productive. It can even help you make more money.

Get the right quality of sleep.

According to the National Sleep Foundation, we all sleep in 90-minute cycles that repeat themselves throughout the night, alternating between REM, or "rapid-eye-movement" and NREM, or "non-rapid-eye-movement" sleep).[47]

When we first fall asleep, we enter the NREM cycle. In the NREM cycle, we move between being awake or lightly sleeping to a drop in body temperature and disengagement from our surroundings, to deep, restorative sleep. During that deep, restorative sleep, our blood pressure drops, breathing becomes slower, muscles are relaxed, blood supply to muscles increases, tissue growth and repair occurs, energy is restored, and hormones are released—such as growth hormone, which is essential for growth and development, including muscle development.[48] NREM generally lasts approximately 75% of the cycle, and night.[49]

From there we move to REM sleep, which lasts about 25% of the cycle and night, during which our brain and body are energized, daytime performance is supported, our brains are active, we dream, our bodies become immobile and relaxed, and our muscles are turned off.[50]

This cycle repeats itself approximately every ninety minutes, resulting in restorative and energizing sleep that sets us up to obtain all the great benefits sleep has to offer.

Follow three guidelines for getting ideal sleep.

It's important that any sleep guidelines not only ensure you can regularly get the right amount of sleep, including avoiding too much sleep,[51] but also ensure you get the right quality of sleep. Although that sounds complicated, like the other N.E.W.S.S.S.S. key areas of life, the ideal amount of sleep can be simplified into a few easy-to-remember guidelines.

First, make sure you get the right amount of sleep. Adults between 18 and 64 years of age should get between seven and nine hours per night, according to the National Sleep Foundation, in association with a multidisciplinary expert panel.[52] For adults who are 65 years old and older, the recommendation is to get between seven and eight hours of sleep a night.[53] This is your general target and ensures that you're getting the right quantity of sleep to avoid the negative health effects associated with sleep deprivation and take advantage of the positive health impacts of sleep.

Second, make sure to structure your evenings to take advantage of the natural sleep aids God built within each of us. God made us, along with nearly all other living organisms, to operate on roughly 24-hour cycles, called our circadian rhythms.

The National Institute of General Medical Sciences describes it as the "physical, mental, and behavioral changes that follow a roughly 24-hour cycle, responding primarily to light and darkness in [our] environment."[54] As light in our environment decreases, our circadian rhythms tell our brain to produce melatonin to prepare our bodies and mind for rest. When light becomes brighter, our circadian rhythms tell our brain to produce less melatonin to wake us up and keep us awake. This results in a natural pattern of higher melatonin production after the sun sets, reaching a point around ten or eleven o'clock at night where most people naturally feel drowsy. If melatonin production is interrupted because of a natural melatonin deficiency that causes our bodies to not produce enough melatonin, or by unnatural interruptions such as excessive blue lights from phone, computer, or TV screens, the cycle God created us to naturally follow gets disrupted and sleep quality and quantity can suffer.

By structuring your evenings to take advantage of your body's natural melatonin production and the circadian rhythms, you will put yourself in a position to fall asleep more easily and stay asleep for the right amount of time.

Finally, make sure to create an environment that promotes good quality sleep. For example, in highlighting what happens when we sleep, the National Sleep Foundation notes that our body temperatures drop naturally during NREM sleep and that, as a result, sleeping in a cooler environment is generally helpful.[55] Additionally, because we know the blue lights from smart phones and other screens interrupt our natural melatonin production, shutting off all screens at least an hour before bedtime is usually helpful.

By following these three guidelines, I've designed a simple sleep plan to help you take advantage of everything we know about sleep to make sure you get the right amount of quality sleep to thrive. This simple sleep plan can form the foundation for a healthy, vibrant, feeling good life.

YOUR SIMPLE SLEEP PLAN

1. Have a scheduled bedtime and wake time, seven days a week, which takes advantage of your natural melatonin production. By doing this you will not only allow your body to get into a rhythm, but you will also make healthy sleep a simple and predictable part of your lifestyle. If you're able to, going to bed around 10:00 p.m. or so allows you to take advantage of your body's natural melatonin production, helping you fall asleep more easily. This can be hard—or impossible—for people who work nights or who have infants or small children, of course, but to the extent possible, commit to a regular bedtime and set your alarm for seven to nine hours later.

2. Engage in moderate physical activity during the day. Moderate exercise has been linked to better sleep, even in patients suffering from insomnia.[56] Do the best you can to get moderate exercise, such as aerobic exercise or even stretching, during the day.

3. Avoid large meals before bedtime. Contrary to popular practice, dinner should be the smallest meal of the day. Having a moderate-sized dinner and waiting at least three hours between eating and your bedtime will generally give your body enough time to digest.

4. Avoid caffeine, alcohol, and nicotine at night. Although some people can have a shot of espresso minutes before falling asleep soundly, caffeine is a stimulant that has been shown to cause insomnia and sleep disturbance.[57] Additionally, while alcohol might make you fall asleep a little faster, studies have shown that drinking alcohol at night can reduce the quality of your sleep, especially if it's done night after night.[58]

Finally, like caffeine, nicotine is a stimulant that has been linked to insomnia and other sleep disturbances.[59]

5. Make sure your bedroom is quiet, dark, relaxing, and not too hot or cold. These environmental factors will help you make sure your bedroom is set up to promote sleep. Some of this can be a challenge if you're married and your spouse is more comfortable with a hotter or colder temperature. My wife, Kim, and I are like this. She's always cold and I'm always hot. One way to reach a compromise is to find a temperature that's not too hot for either of you and for the person who likes it warmer to use an extra blanket or comforter so each of you can be comfortable throughout the night.

6. Turn all screens off at least an hour before bedtime. We know screens keep your brain running and block melatonin production. As long as that bright light comes into your eyes, your brain won't think it's bedtime and, thus, won't produce the melatonin you need to go to sleep, so shut those screens off at least an hour before bedtime and record any shows you'll miss so you can watch them the next day.

7. Use the restroom right before bed. This will help you make it through the night without waking up to use the restroom.

8. Make your bed as comfortable as possible. I always tell people to get the most comfortable bed they can afford. If you're spending a third of your life—and an important third of your life—on one piece of furniture, making sure you're comfortable and getting the full mental, emotional, and physical health benefits from it is key. You're investing in your overall health by investing in a new, comfortable bed,

so be sure to get the most comfortable bed possible for your budget. If your bed is old, saggy, or just uncomfortable, then buying a new, comfortable bed will help you get to sleep more easily and stay asleep better throughout the night.

OPTIMAL LIVING ACTION STEPS

1. Commit to building healthy sleep habits.

2. Calculate the time you need to get up in the morning to make it to work. Set your alarm for that time and count back seven to nine hours if you're between 18 and 64 years old. Commit to that time being your bedtime for the next seven days, aiming for a bedtime around 10:00 p.m. At the very least, have a more consistent bedtime and wake time.

3. Unplug all electronics in your room and shut down anything with a screen at least an hour before bedtime. Lower the lights in your house around that time as well to let your body begin to relax and produce melatonin.

4. During the last hour, take a shower and brush your teeth so you feel relaxed and refreshed.

5. Wear the same comfortable clothes to bed routinely. If you can, try sleeping without clothes, which according to several recent studies has been associated with regulating your body temperature and getting deeper, longer sleep, as well as giving you other health benefits.[60] [61]

6. Write down anything you need to do the next day before you go to bed so you aren't thinking about it when you're trying to fall asleep.

7. Turn on a fan or calming white noise to prevent outside noises from waking you up.

8. Consider having a stress assessment done. If you've had issues with stress in your life, either currently or in the past, I suggest you look into having an adrenal stress assessment done. The stress could have disrupted your circadian rhythm and could be the underlying cause to your sleep issues. To learn more about having a stress assessment done, visit HowToLiveUntilYouDie.com

Chapter 5

SUPPLEMENTS

How to Find the Supplements Your Body Needs and Avoid the Chemicals it Doesn't

"One of the biggest tragedies of human civilization is the precedents of chemical therapy over nutrition. It's a substitution of artificial therapy over nature, of poisons over food, in which we are feeding people poisons trying to correct the reactions of starvation."

– Dr. Royal Lee

EVERYTHING WE NEED TO provide the nutrients we require for all kinds of functions in our body, we should be getting from food. That's where we should be getting our nutrition. There are vitamins and minerals in food that our bodies require for all sorts of functions.

God made food loaded with these nutrients that we have to have for our bodies to work like He designed them to work. He told us, in Genesis 1:29, "Behold, I have given you every plant yielding seed that is on the surface of all the earth, and every tree which has fruit yielding seed; it shall be food for you." So why do we need supplements, then?

If you're like most people, when it comes to supplements, you want your supplement intake to be minimal, easy to take, and effective. The problem many people have with supplements is not knowing what supplements to take, if any. They don't know what they need, how much of it they need, and why they need it.

Supplements are often thought of as expensive compared to $4 generic drug copay options. When people consider supplements, it's easy to get confused by so many options. From pills to powders, all-in-one multivitamins to individual nutrients, the possibilities are endless. Additionally, because the supplement market isn't nearly as regulated as the prescription or over-the-counter drug market, it's hard to know exactly what's in each supplement.

Moreover, it is quicker and easier to mask symptoms (which many prescription drugs do very well) than it is to resolve nutrient deficiencies in the body (which supplements tend to do well). Therefore, people tend to view prescription drugs as more effective than supplements because drugs often quickly mask symptoms even though they may not always be the long-term cure to the underlying issue, which in some cases requires a longer commitment to nutrient supplementation or lifestyle changes. Due to this, supplements are frequently looked at as "snake oil," or something only "health nuts" believe in. People rationalize, *if that natural herb really solved the problem, everyone would just eat vegetables and nobody would be suffering.*

I understand those frustrations. I experienced them myself, too. I've taken hundreds of supplements in my life. Some of those supplements worked well, but others didn't. I've felt the "quick fix" from a drug masking symptoms only to have the same problem over and over again because the underlying problem wasn't solved.

I've also studied supplements and nutrition for over two decades. I've learned what makes a supplement a "good" supplement and what makes it a "bad" supplement. Over that time, I've discovered that looking at the price tag or the popularity of a supplement is one of the worst ways to choose one because the value of a supplement is not how many pills per dollar you're receiving, but how much of a benefit you're receiving from taking those supplements.

Finally, and most importantly, I've learned how to know whether you need to take supplements and, if so, what supplements to take first, and how to measure whether they are helping you.

Although Michel de Montaigne famously said, "There is no knowledge so hard to acquire as the knowledge of how to live this life well and naturally," my goal with this information is to make the process of acquiring information about living well and naturally easier and simpler than ever before. Thus, I wrote this chapter with that in mind. This information can help you make better-informed choices about your health and which natural options are available to you.

Do you need to take supplements?

Supplements, like the name implies, are only needed to supplement our diet. If we get everything we need from food, we don't need vitamins.

There is no substitute for getting our nutrients from real food. Unfortunately, it's not always possible to get all the nutrients our bodies require from *real* food. Over the past several decades, although the quantity of food in developed countries has increased, the quality of the food has diminished exponentially. What most people eat these days isn't God-made food, but rather man-made food that's genetically modified or full of toxins. Much of that food might fill your stomach, but it's also devoid of nutrients.

Because of that, many medical professionals find that people need to augment their nutrition with *some* level of supplements to make sure they're getting the right nutrients in the right amounts.

What kind of supplements should you take?

Walk into any drug store and you'll see rows of vitamins and supplements of all different types. Choose the right one and, over time, you can vastly improve your health and nutrient composition by giving your body the nutrients it lacks and nothing more. Choose the wrong one and you might as well swallow the $10 bill you wasted on a child-proof bottle of pills full of artificial colors, flavors, dyes, and fillers.

In fact, you might be shocked to find artificial colors, flavors, preservatives, and other Big Seven Toxins in many of the multivitamins that you've been told are a one-pill-per-day solution. In reality, many of those vitamins are a waste of your time and money.

Fortunately, it's relatively simple to avoid wasting your money on ineffective or toxin-filled vitamins by simply looking at the label and following three simple guidelines. Although it may take a few minutes to find supplements that fit these guidelines, you generally only need to do it once. Once you find the right supplements, you know exactly what to buy going forward.

There is no substitute for getting our nutrients from real food.

First, avoid the same dangerous chemicals and ingredients that you would avoid in food and look instead for ingredients that are organic or substances found in nature.

Second, avoid toxic coatings and unhealthy binders like soybean oil, titanium dioxide, or sodium selenite that are found in many multivitamins, which your body will often not recognize. Instead, look for plant-based binders such as microcrystalline cellulose, hydroxypropyl cellulose, arrowroot, croscarmellose sodium, or silica.

Finally, ask your pharmacist or health-care provider about options that list all of the vitamins and nutrients in milligrams because that can be an indication that the product is synthetic and doesn't contain food-sourced nutrients. In some cases, the vitamin and nutrient content of natural foods varies too much to be that precise, so ask your pharmacist or health-care provider whether the nutrients are sourced from food.

If you need help with this, feel free to contact me at HowToLiveUntilYouDie.com.

In summary, you should generally avoid these:

- Ingredients with names you don't know as healthy and can't pronounce.
- Any kinds of dye, like "Red 40," "Yellow 6," etc.
- Dangerous binders like soybean oil, titanium dioxide, or sodium selenite.
- Chemical coating, like phthalates or polyvinyl alcohol.

Instead, look for these:

- Ingredients with names of substances found in nature.
- Vitamins that contain at least some organic ingredients.
- Plant-based binders like microcrystalline cellulose, hydroxypropyl cellulose, arrowroot, croscarmellose sodium; no toxic coating.

By following these guidelines, you will end up with a much higher-quality vitamin made from natural ingredients without toxic chemicals that you wouldn't want to put in your body.

Although you'll likely find that the natural supplements are a little more expensive than the ones that are full of toxic chemicals, you can rest assured that the money you spent was on natural ingredients and not for the privilege of eating little pills of chemicals. That extra cost is a wise investment in my book.

If you're still unsure about a particular supplement,

you can contact the company and ask for what's called an "independent assay" of the ingredients.

An independent assay is a test conducted by an independent third party to determine exactly what's in the supplement. Many natural-supplement companies will have independent assays conducted of their products and proudly send them to you.

If a company you're considering can't or won't give you an independent assay of their product, it doesn't necessarily mean they can't be trusted, but because there are so many supplement companies that have them available, it's easier to stick with one that can prove the content of their products to you.

What supplement company can you trust?

Because the supplement industry isn't as regulated as prescription or over-the-counter medications, it's hard to know what companies you can trust. This makes label reading important, especially to look for ingredients to avoid, so you can at least narrow down your options to the vitamins that appear, from their labels, to be healthy.

From there, the most reliable way to make a decision is to do a few more minutes of research into the reputation and track record of the company. Even a simple Google search about the company will likely give you company history, consumer complaints and reviews, and testimonials. Look at their websites and see how long they've been around and where they source their products from.

Determine your vitamin or nutrient deficiencies.

Millions of people have vitamin or nutrient deficiencies that can lead to significant and debilitating conditions like anemia, diabetes, osteoporosis, depression, and even cancer, and they don't even know it. Many of these people experience symptoms like feeling tired or weak, gaining weight, or having aches and pains.

Other people don't display any symptoms or are so used to the symptoms that they don't even notice that they're on their way to a significant health condition. Sometimes people can correct these problems by taking supplements or adjusting their diet, but they never do because they don't know.

Many deficiencies can be identified in the blood tests that are typically done at our annual physicals. One of the blood tests, called a CBC, or complete blood count, can return information about anemia, B12 deficiencies, folic acid deficiencies, or iron deficiencies. Those are all nutrients found in food and supplements.

They also sometimes run a CMP, or comprehensive metabolic panel, blood test. The CMP looks at organ function to check for conditions like diabetes, liver disease, or kidney diseases, as well as electrolytes in your body (your minerals: sodium, potassium, chloride, and calcium). There's also one mineral—magnesium—that is often not a part of the standard metabolic panel, and only checked by request, which I encourage you to do.

To find out what other tests you can take either independently or at your next physical to ensure you have broad information about potential deficiencies, download a list of suggested tests on the resources page at HowToLiveUntilYouDie.com.

Your test results often do a decent job of explaining recommended levels for each nutrient or vitamin they measure, so you can tell if you're deficient in something. If you're right in the middle of a healthy range, you're probably okay. If you start getting toward the end of a range, I suggest talking with someone specifically about that for advice.

Once you get the results of your tests, going over the results with your physician or another professional will help you identify what you might need to get more of through your food consumption or a good supplement. This will help you identify things that are unique to your measurements for you to take. They'll also make sure you don't take supplements that don't work well together or that might cause a negative reaction with a medication you take.

What about all of your prescriptions?

The point of this information is not to tell you to throw out all of your prescription medications. In fact, many people need traditional medications to survive. The point of this chapter is twofold.

First, it's designed to share information about how to choose high-quality supplements so you can make better-informed choices when evaluating supplements.

Second, it's designed to give you more information about natural additions or alternatives to discuss with your healthcare provider in order to consider whether natural supplements might be useful in your unique situation, either in addition to or instead of some of your prescription medications. This could be on a regular basis, like with daily vitamin supplementation, or in response to specific symptoms or conditions you experience.

For example, a client of mine, Dan Miller, author of the *New York Times* Bestselling book, *48 Days to the Work You Love*, came to me after finishing a big push to promote his latest book, *Wisdom Meets Passion*. Dan had coached me through growing my natural pharmacy and health-and-wellness coaching and consulting practice, so he was very familiar with me.

One of the things that Dan appreciated about my practice was that I was a traditionally trained pharmacist and, in his words, "working to get people off the medication I was selling," if we could determine there were natural alternatives that were just as good or better for them.

Dan was struggling with fatigue, low energy, irritability, digestive problems, and even chest pains at night. At first, he was convinced that he was just burned out after a decade of exponential business growth and a recent book launch, so he went to his primary-care doctor. Because of the chest pain, his health-care provider sent him to a cardiologist to conduct a stress test to investigate whether Dan was suffering from a serious heart condition.

The stress test confirmed that Dan's heart was strong, so his health-care providers believed his low energy, irritability, and fatigue were caused by burnout and his digestive problems and chest pains were the result of reflux. Based on that evaluation, Dan was told to slow down and take Omeprazole, a medication to decrease the amount of acid his stomach produces, for the rest of his life to manage his physical discomfort.

When Dan approached me with his symptoms and doctor's suggested treatment, I agreed that Dan was displaying all the symptoms of burnout. However, like many conditions, I knew that those same symptoms could be caused by many things, not just burnout, so I suggested that Dan take a simple DNA analysis and adrenal stress test to evaluate his hormone levels, digestive system health, and other issues.

The DNA analysis and adrenal stress test revealed

that Dan had imbalances within his body that could be addressed by natural supplements and other simple lifestyle adjustments, primarily concerning sleep patterns, so he might not need to be taking Omeprazole. Dan continued to work with his health-care provider as we started working natural supplements into his routine based on what his body told us through the DNA analysis and adrenal stress test.

Over time, Dan's symptoms disappeared. His sleep improved. His energy skyrocketed. And his body felt better than it had in years.

What changed? As with everything I offer in this book, Dan and I focused on getting more information about his body and the underlying issue, and not just eliminating big issues like heart disease and then managing symptoms. Traditional medication is skewed toward managing symptoms, so the natural reaction from his physicians was to prescribe rest and traditional medications for the symptoms.

Instead, Dan invested less than four hundred dollars to conduct a complete analysis of his body so we could identify deficiencies to resolve, instead of only symptoms to treat. In doing so, we discovered natural solutions to Dan's discomfort, restored balance within Dan's body, and resolved the underlying issue through probiotics and digestive enzymes.

What are the five most commonly needed supplements?

In addition to responding to specific conditions or symptoms, like Dan's experience, natural supplementation can be beneficial as alternatives to synthetic supplements on a regular basis, too. Unless you're eating only organic, homegrown foods, there is a good chance that you need some general supplementation because your food will likely not be able to provide you enough vitamins or minerals.

Over the past few decades, most people I've encountered have discovered that they could benefit from at least one of the five most commonly needed supplements. These supplements are so commonly needed and beneficial that I take each of these on a daily basis myself.

The vitamin I recommend for most of my clients is a high-quality general multivitamin. From a quality perspective, I've found that virtually all of the multivitamins you see in the big box stores contain at least one of the Big Seven Toxins. The multivitamin that I prefer, and take myself, is called Catalyn by Standard Process. Catalyn has been on the market since 1929 and is made from organic foods grown on an organic-only farm in Wisconsin.

Another supplement that I find beneficial for most people is a high-quality fish oil, which may help promote brain function and prevent Alzheimer's Disease. It also acts as an anti-inflammatory, which has several additional health benefits like promoting neurological health and supporting mood and memory. The one I take myself and recommend is ProDHA by Nordic Naturals, which is sourced from the cold, Icelandic waters of Norway. If you cannot take fish oil for some reason, krill oil might be an option, as it has many of the same benefits of fish oil.

A third supplement that I find most people could benefit from is a high-quality probiotic, which restores to the body the natural bacteria that get depleted from eating too many processed foods or taking common medications like antibiotics and steroids. As with all supplements, you could get the necessary amount of bacteria from eating foods like real yogurt, tofu, sauerkraut, or unpasteurized, unprocessed butter on a daily basis.

If you're not eating foods rich in those natural bacteria, a high-quality probiotic might be just what you need because the natural bacteria is a vital part of our immune system that performs several important functions in our bodies, including protecting us from disease.

With probiotics, it's important that you choose one that needs to be refrigerated, because that tells you it has live versions of the bacteria, which will serve your body best. If it's shelf stable, it means that the bacteria may be dead and less helpful. The one I take is called Enterbiotic SBO by Natural Creations, which is dairy-, soy-, dye-, and gluten-free. Another one I recommend often is Primal Defense by Garden of Life.

Fourth, a vitamin I've found the majority of my clients deficient in is Vitamin D. Optimal Vitamin D levels are between 50 and 80 ng/mL. Between 30 and 50 ng/mL is considered low. Below 30 ng/mL is deficient. Vitamin D deficiency can lead to an increased risk of death from cardiovascular disease, cognitive impairment for older adults, severe asthma in children, and cancer. Nationwide, millions of people suffer from Vitamin D deficiency.

The most effective way to naturally get Vitamin D is to get outside with exposed skin for about 30 minutes between 11:00 a.m. and 2:00 p.m. If you're not getting enough exposure to the sun on a daily basis, it's possible that you are Vitamin D deficient. If you can't add that sunlight into your schedule, I highly suggest taking a quality Vitamin D supplement on a daily basis. Your health-care provider can tell you what dose to take based on your recent blood work. If you have any questions, please feel free to reach out to me at HowToLiveUntilYouDie.com.

Finally, I also often recommend Coenzyme Q10, or CoQ10, which as you know from Jerry's story, is a naturally occurring enzyme in our body and good for heart health. I especially recommend it to people taking a cholesterol-lowering statin drug, as those drugs deplete the levels of CoQ10 in our bodies. My favorite CoQ10 product is Smart CoQ10 by Enzymatic Therapy, because it's a quality supplement that's chewable, which allows it to be absorbed more readily.

Is it a miracle solution?

Dan's experience demonstrates the value of considering alternative testing and treatment in addition to traditional medicine; however, it's important to remember that I'm not encouraging anyone to ignore traditional medicine altogether. I'm not suggesting that natural supplements are the miracle cure to all problems. What I teach about supplements works best in conjunction with traditional medicine. My goal is to help you become more informed, to give you additional information to discuss with your health-care providers so you can find the best solution for you.

My goal for any supplement or medication regime is to address the underlying problem, not just treat the symptoms. The goal is to be healthy and keep your body working well. Sometimes, the best solution for you will be a traditional prescription. There's nothing wrong with that if it's the appropriate response to your condition. Other times, however, traditional prescription medications will be ineffective or will only treat the symptoms of your condition, instead of actually resolving your condition. A natural supplement might be the best route for you when that is the case.

Still other times, you may find that making adjustments to one or more of the other N.E.W.S.S.S.S. key areas of life is your solution. Supplements are just one part of a balanced plan to become happy, healthy, and whole.

By being informed about these seven key areas of life, including natural options for nutrition and supplements, you can be better prepared to work with your health-care providers to find the right solution for you.

OPTIMAL LIVING ACTION STEPS

1. Go to HowToLiveUntilYouDie.com to get a list of blood tests and result information.

2. Reach out to your physician or another professional to help you analyze recent test results.

3. If you haven't had blood work recently, consider scheduling it with your physician or having it conducted on the private market. You can get many tests done for a pretty reasonable out-of-pocket cost if you don't have insurance to pay for it. The value of the information to your health is well worth it.

4. Consider picking up a good multivitamin, fish or krill oil, and a probiotic like the ones mentioned here or at HowToLiveUntilYouDie.com, which are ones I've taken or at least researched myself. If you know you are or think you could be Vitamin D deficient, consider picking up a good Vitamin D supplement as well. If you're taking a cholesterol-lowering statin drug, consider picking up some Coenzyme Q10.

5. Finally, consider obtaining a mail-in genetic analysis that will tell you what specific supplements you may need to take based upon your diet and DNA. Like I mentioned before, many of the tests even come with customized nutrition and exercise information to help you choose the best foods and exercise routines for your body. You can learn more about DNA testing at HowToLiveUntilYouDie.com.

Right: My six blessings...
our five plus Madison,
our Daughter-in-Law.

Below: Our big
happy, healthy and
whole family on
Christmas Day 2015.

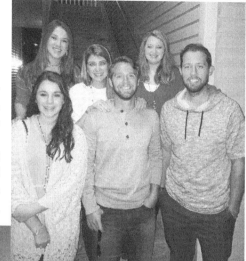

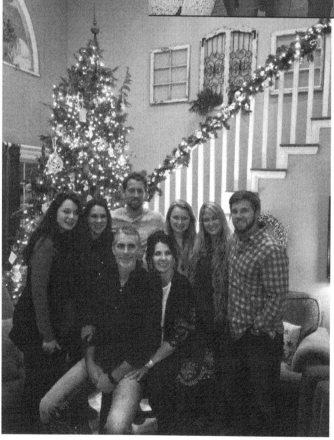

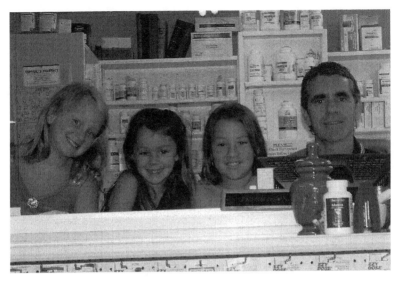

My three little girls helping me out in the pharmacy, Fall 2005.

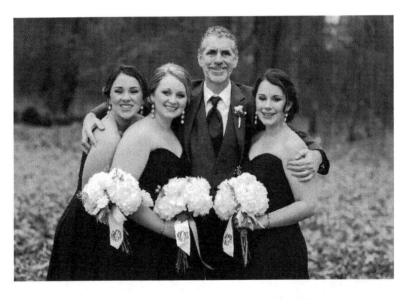

Me and my girls on Cody and Madison's wedding day.
Beautiful girls inside and out.

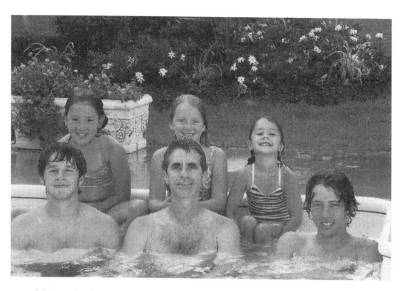

Me and all my cubs enjoying the pool on Father's Day 2005.

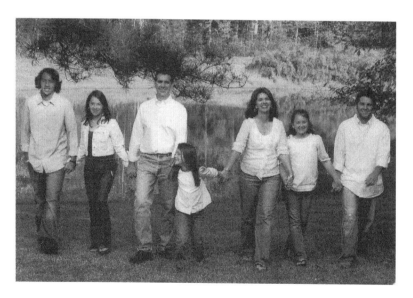

One of our last family photos taken
before they all started flying the coop.

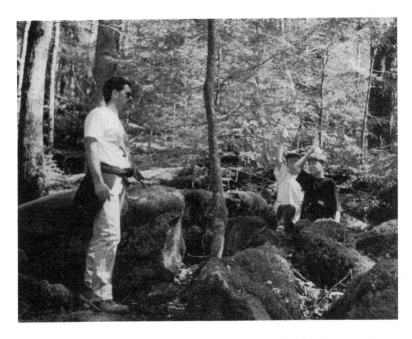

Above: Me and the two boys on a hiking trip in the Smoky Mountains. One of our favorite things to do with the kids when they were growing up.

Right: Me and my two boys preparing for soccer season in 2005. Soccer was a big part of our lives for many years.

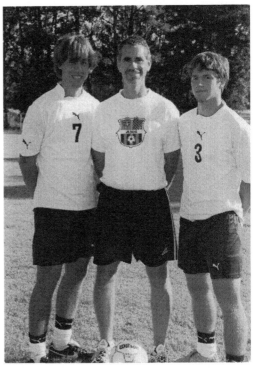

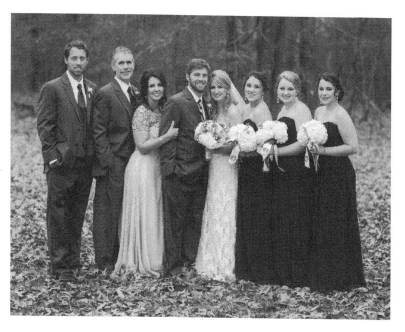

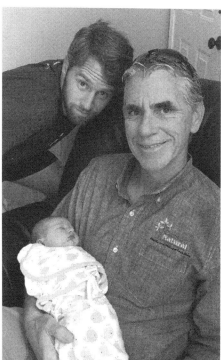

Above: Cody and Madison's wedding day 12/13/14.

Left: Three generations of firstborns. Myself, my firstborn son, Cody, and my firstborn grandchild, Charlee.

Right: University of Mississippi School of Pharmacy graduation day, May 1985.

Below: Kim and I leaving the Church on our Wedding Day 3/10/1984. We had no idea the amazing journey that was ahead for us.

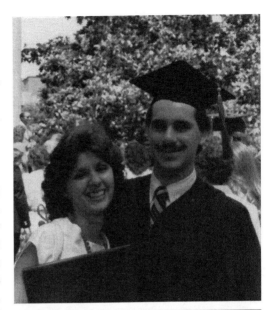

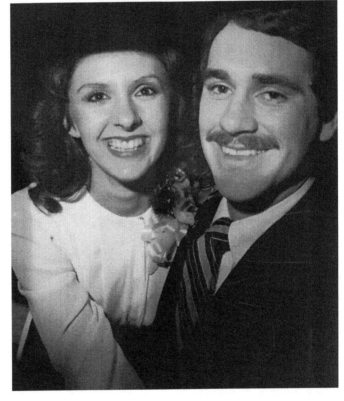

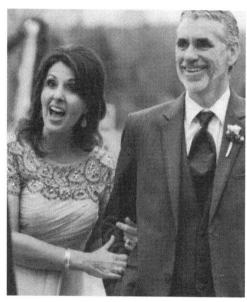

Left: A joyous moment for Kim and I on Cody and Madison's wedding day.

Below: Our kids favorite picture of Kim and I, taken during some tough times. Kim has always been able to find Joy in the Journey.

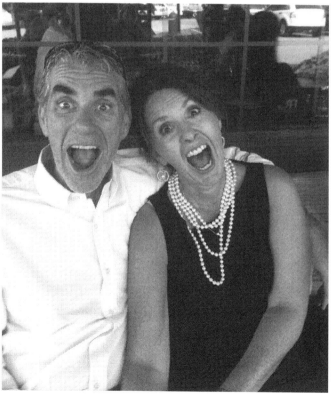

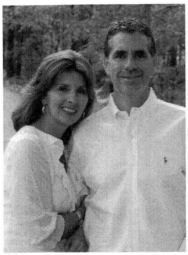

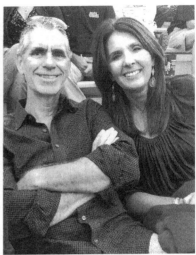

Top Left: Kim
and I doing a
photo shoot on
our property
in 2007. Happy
days before life's
storms of 2008
and 2009 hit.

Top Right: Kim
and I enjoying
game day at Ole
Miss, Oct 2015.

Right: Kim
and I enjoying
New York City
Christmas 2014.

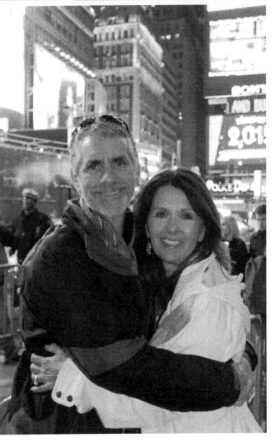

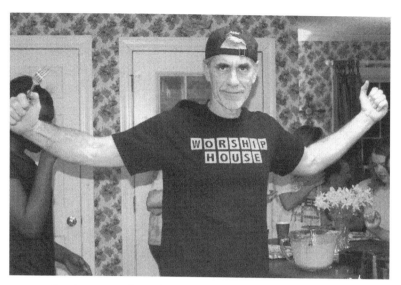

Serving one of our favorite meals, gluten-free protein
waffles to all the kids in our church youth group.
Best waffles ever is what they all say.

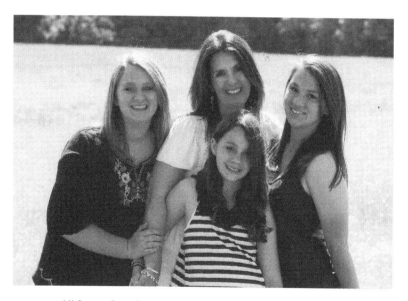

All four of my beautiful girls. This pic was taken in a
meadow near our property in the Spring of 2011. I am
extremely blessed to be continually surrounded by beauty.

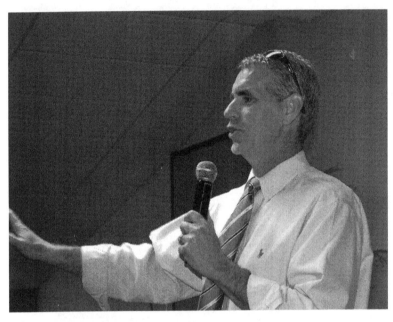

Love to take every opportunity I get to speak and spread the message of natural health and wellness.

CHAPTER 6
SOUL

How and Why to Find Peace of Mind and Emotional Peace

"He has achieved success who has lived well, laughed often, and loved much."

— Bessie A. Stanley

STUDIES HAVE FOUND THAT stress levels are at an all-time high and the effects of stress are debilitating and widespread. Too many people live in a state of constant worry with deep emotional scars that they've carried around for years.

On a day-to-day basis, all the family and work obligations leave people exhausted and without any time or energy left for themselves. From a broader perspective, people feel out of control, with kids who won't listen, bosses who don't understand, and economic or geopolitical environments that create panic and fear.

All that stress is taking a physical and emotional toll on people, causing or exacerbating high blood pressure, general unhappiness, anxiety, depression, and even physical symptoms like aches and pains, headaches, digestive issues, stomachaches, dizziness, vomiting, and weight gain.[62]

Too many people live in a state of constant worry with deep emotional scars that they've carried around for years.

I struggled with stress and soul sickness for decades. I grew up in a stressful, even dysfunctional home. The only positive thoughts and emotions I experienced were a matter of choice and faith because they weren't part of my natural environment.

As an adult, I experienced extended bouts of stress and pain. In 2009, my wife Kim and I went through an incredibly challenging time financially. We lost nearly everything but our house. It was tough. I felt like I had no control and only one way out, which was to choose positive thoughts and emotions and run closer to God. We both did. We got through that time because of our faith in God, because we went closer to God, and because we had each other.

We ran to Him, not away from Him. Many nights on my prayer walks, I'd walk up and down the road confessing to God that "I am happy, healthy, and whole, happy, healthy, and whole." To the outside world, and even in my own mind, I was depressed, heartsick, and *in a hole*—a big hole—but I confessed to God, and I put my faith in God, that He would make us happy, healthy, and whole.

Therefore humble yourselves under the mighty hand of God, that He may exalt you in due time, casting all your care upon Him, for He cares for you.
– 1 Peter 5:6-7 (NKJV)

The more time I spent with God telling Him that we were happy, healthy, and whole, the more I felt God leading me away from the stress, from focusing on the parts of my life that I couldn't control, and toward healing and happiness and making better choices in matters I could control.

Over the next six years, we made choices and took actions that we never would have done without our faith and support and the intentional choice to confess, to profess to God that we were happy, healthy, and whole. For example, many people's initial reaction to tough financial times is to close up, to cut charitable endeavors, and spend all their time and money within the four walls of their homes. We decided, however, to continue to give both money and our time throughout those tough times, even though we were dangerously close to going bankrupt. We gave to our church, our community, and others.

We also made forgiveness a priority. I, for example, let go of the guilt and shame I felt for being in the financial mess. I chose to forgive everyone whom I had carried ill will toward in my heart, some for as far back in time as my childhood, and cleared all the negative emotions from my heart. By doing so, my heart became full of my faith in God and my love for my family, friends, and community. That mental and emotional shift was transformational.

Although there were many painful nights, we experienced tremendous growth, love, and peace during that time. Today, we're both happy, healthy, and whole. We've been married over thirty-two years. We continue to actively serve our church and community, have five adult kids who are doing well, and we even became grandparents. We have peace of mind and emotional peace. Our souls are strong, and our hearts are full of faith and love.

Soul sickness can have physical manifestations.

A client of mine, whom I'll call Jim to protect his identity, had a similarly transformational experience after he worked through a soul sickness that had stuck with him for years. "Jim" has given me permission to share his story with you to demonstrate the powerful, positive effect a healthy soul can have on your life; however, we both agree that utilizing a pseudonym for him is wise.

Jim came to me in a lot of physical and emotional pain. His father had struggled with a pornography addiction for most of Jim's life. No matter how much Jim or his mother tried to help his father overcome the addiction, nothing worked and his parents ultimately divorced when Jim was a teenager. Unfortunately, Jim also struggled with a pornography addiction of his own from the time he was a teenager until he was into his early thirties.

Even after being freed from his addiction upon his baptism and finding Christ, Jim continued to struggle with his thoughts, emotions, and lustful urges for years, although he was able to resist acting upon those urges. At the same time, Jim suffered from severe back pain that he couldn't overcome despite seeking treatment from many doctors and chiropractors and engaging in years of stretching, strengthening, and chiropractic treatments.

When Jim shared his history of pain, addiction, and spiritual awakening with me, I recognized the deep pain he was experiencing, not only in his back, but also in his heart. Even though he got past his addiction, he continued to struggle with his father's leaving and his lustful urges, so we explored how he could work on his soul sickness to alleviate his guilt and pain. I recommended he read a book called *The Ties That Bind*, by my friend Brian Holmes. In the book, Brian discusses how many people have unresolved issues from past relationships, events, or experiences that wreak havoc in their lives, and helps the reader address and resolve those issues so they can experience the abundant life that God has always intended for them.

> *"The calm and balanced mind*
> *is the strong and great mind;*
> *the hurried and agitated mind*
> *is the weak one."*
> **– Wallace D. Wattles**

After applying the lessons Brian shares in the book, Jim began a transformation that reached beyond his wildest expectations. He realized that his pain, feelings, and addictions traced back to his experience with his father and was able to finally address those issues at their core. By doing so, his lustful desires disappeared, his guilt and shame evaporated, and the debilitating back pain he suffered from for decades was no more.

Jim now lives a pain-, guilt-, and shame-free life because he went beyond his body and dug deep into his soul, and serves as a great example of how unresolved soul sickness can be part or all of the reason for physical pain, not just emotional issues.

Guard your soul.

This chapter can do the same for you as it did for Jim, Kim, and me. This chapter can help you cleanse your soul, removing the negative, stressful, heavy baggage from your heart. In doing so, you will improve your outlook on life, the quality of your sleep, your relationships with family, friends, and coworkers, and even your self-esteem. Your heart can be full of faith and love, and you can begin to feel happy, healthy, and whole, deep in your soul.

Proverbs 4:23 tells us to "Keep your heart with all diligence. For out of it *spring* the issues of life." (NKJV) In the New Living Translation of the same verse, we're directed to "Guard your heart above all else, for it determines the course of your life."

Although both versions of this Scripture utilize the old English version of the word "heart," we know that the word "heart" translates to today's language as "soul." Moreover, when we experience the pain and stress of a wounded soul, we often feel it right in our hearts.

In other words, the Bible tells us to guard our souls above all else because it determines the course of our lives.

It doesn't matter how strong or healthy our bodies are, if our hearts—or our souls—are full of pain and stress, we can't be whole. That's why He tells us to guard our hearts, to be diligent in keeping our hearts full of faith and love and not guilt, shame, and pain.

> **Your heart can be full of faith and love, and you can begin to feel happy, healthy, and whole, deep in your soul.**

The challenge with that exercise is that there's no objective test to determine what you need to let go of, whom you need to forgive, and what thoughts you need to counteract, regarding your soul. There's no blood test, bathroom scale, or step counter to tell you how healthy your soul is.

The only measures we have are our minds and our hearts. Those are God's tools for measuring and improving our soul health. Our minds can tell us what negative thoughts or emotions we're holding and help us choose to let go. Our hearts are where we store the pain or joy of our souls. When our souls are suffering, our hearts feel heavy. When our souls are healed, we literally feel our hearts lighten. We feel peace in our hearts.

Thus, the first step in cleansing your soul involves recognizing that your soul is an integral part of who you are and what you become, which affects your body and your spirit. Your soul, while felt in your heart, is a separate part of who you are, independent from your physical body.

"Most people fail at whatever they attempt because of an undecided heart. Should I? Should I not? Go forward? Go back? Success requires the emotional balance of a committed heart. When confronted with a challenge, the committed heart will search for a solution. The undecided heart searches for an escape. A committed heart does not wait for conditions to be exactly right. Why? Because conditions are never exactly right. Indecision limits the Almighty and His ability to perform miracles in your life. He has put the vision in you – proceed. To wait, to wonder, to doubt, to be indecisive is to disobey God."

– Andy Andrews,
The Traveler's Gift

The next step in cleansing your soul is to spend a few minutes in quiet each day listening to what your heart is telling you. What negative thoughts, emotions, or feelings are you holding in there? What do you feel guilty about?

What are you shameful for? Is there someone you haven't forgiven? Is there someone you need to apologize to? What negative thoughts do you feel about yourself?

The answers to these questions will lead you to the next step in cleansing your soul, which is to begin taking steps to release the negative mental and emotional pain you're carrying in your heart. This involves making a choice to let go of those negative feelings.

For example, you may be carrying guilt or shame in your heart because you wronged someone years ago and may need to sincerely apologize to them for it. By sincerely apologizing to people you've wronged, you will have taken every step within your control to right those wrongs and release those negative thoughts and emotions, even if the person isn't ready to accept your apology. They may never accept your apology, or they may at a later date, but by sincerely recognizing and apologizing for wrongs you've committed, you're taking the first step to clearing the guilt and shame you've been carrying in your heart.

True forgiveness is a powerful way to improve the health of your soul.

Similarly, you may be carrying pain in your heart because somebody wronged you and you may need to choose to forgive them, even if they don't believe they've done anything wrong. By doing so, you'll be taking the first step to clearing the pain you've been carrying in your heart. True forgiveness is a powerful way to improve the health of your soul. It's been linked to several positive mental and physical health benefits, including even assisting with immune function and fighting cancer.[63] One important note about forgiveness to remember is that forgiveness doesn't take place in your words; it takes place in your heart and mind. In fact, you can begin a process of forgiveness without even letting the person who wronged you know that you forgive them. You can forgive them in your mind and heart and just let go of the pain.

So many people are sick today because they are carrying around mental and emotional pain in their hearts. They're walking around with heavy anxiety, with wounded hearts—with wounded souls—because somebody has done something to them and they haven't healed those emotional wounds, because they have wronged someone and live with guilt and shame, or because they don't have a strong emotional connection with family, friends, or their community.

By making a decision to walk closer to God, to our families, and our communities; letting go of the pain, guilt, and shame we all hold in our hearts; and giving our time and money to causes we care about, we can cleanse our souls of the negative thoughts and emotions that keep us stressed and depressed, and begin to fill our souls with peace and love.

Getting Help

Soul sickness is not something to take lightly because the issues that people carry around in their souls are often serious and can be debilitating. Because of that, I highly recommend getting help from a trained professional such as a pastor, counselor, or professional coach. There's plenty of help available to you, so you don't need to feel like you need to resolve such serious issues on your own. Some people are ready to address these issues, but need help from someone trained and knowledgeable to go deeper than many of us can, or are willing to, do alone.

There are thousands of Christian counselors and coaches who can help you identify and resolve issues that are weighing on your soul. For example, the Professional Christian Coaching Institute, which is run by my good friend Chris McCluskey, has trained thousands of coaches over more than a decade and maintains a directory of Christian coaches throughout the world. The directory is free to search. If you want help finding a Christian coach to walk with you as you continue your health journey, I highly recommend starting with the Professional Christian Coaching Institute and searching the Christian coaches directory. You can find information for both the Professional Christian Coaching Institute and the Christian coaches directory at HowToLiveUntilYouDie.com.

OPTIMAL LIVING ACTION STEPS

1. Answer these nine questions and give yourself one point if the answer is yes. If you accumulate five points, your soul is likely in pretty good shape.

   - Am I at peace with everyone in my life?
   - Have I forgiven everyone who has wronged me in my past?
   - Am I active in a faith community?
   - Do I like spending time with my family?
   - Do I have people in my life who love me as I am?
   - Do I believe my future is going to be positive and healthy?
   - Do I feel in control of my emotions?
   - Do I fall asleep and stay asleep with no trouble?
   - Have I laughed in the past week?

2. Spend fifteen minutes evaluating each question you didn't get a point for in part one and what negative emotion you might need to let go. For example:

   - Do you need to apologize to someone?
   - Do you need to forgive someone?
   - Do you need to give more time or money?
   - Why don't you like spending time with your family? Do you need to spend less time with someone and more time with others?
   - What people in your life don't love you as you are? Do you need to spend less (or no) time with them?
   - Why don't you feel your future is going to be positive or healthy? What can you do differently to be more positive or healthy?
   - Why don't you feel you're in control of your emotions?

- What thoughts or emotions keep you up at night or wake you up in the night?

- For any of these, what obstacles do you face in attempting to let go of the negative emotion? What are two ways you might be able to overcome those options?

3. Take one or two small steps to begin letting go of the negative pain or emotions in your heart. If you're having trouble deciding, I suggest choosing to give time or money to your local church or forgiving someone who has wronged you, because giving and forgiving are perhaps two of the most powerful cures for soul sickness.

4. Spend time working laughter and fun into your daily routine. The Bible tells us that "A cheerful heart is good medicine" in Proverbs 17:22 (NIV). Some of my favorite things to do to incorporate laughter into my life are to watch clean stand-up comedy either live or on YouTube, such as my friend Ken Davis' hilarious materials. You can find links to several of my favorite videos as well as more information about the benefit of laughter, on the resources page at HowToLiveUntilYouDie.com.

Enjoy your days. Laugh. Dance. Smile. Love. These emotions are some of the most important elements of a life worth living. So laugh every day and follow the advice of William W. Purkey, to "Dance like there's nobody watching, Love like you'll never be hurt, Sing like there's nobody listening, And live like it's heaven on earth."

5. Get help if you need it. Get a copy of *The Ties That Bind* by Brian Holmes and work through the lessons Brian teaches. For more individualized help, reach out to a pastor, counselor, or professional

coach to help you go deeper to identify and resolve issues that are causing any soul sickness. For links to the Professional Christian Coaching Institute and its Christian coaches directory, visit HowToLiveUntilYouDie.com.

CHAPTER 7
SPIRIT

Tapping into a Higher Power for Lasting Happiness

"God gave us the gift of life; it is up to us to give ourselves the gift of living well."

— Voltaire

AS THREE-PART BEINGS, WE can have great physical health and internal peace and still feel unbalanced or like we're not tapping into our true potential. That's because the third part of how God made us is the most important part, the glue that holds us together and keeps us happy, healthy, and whole. Spiritual health gives us hope and strength. It gives us power. Yet when it comes to thinking of our overall health, many people give very little thought to the health of their spirit. Because of that, many people struggle with their spiritual health and never achieve the balanced health and happiness that God created each of us to achieve.

> *"To seek the highest good*
> *is to live well."*
> **– St. Augustine**

People struggle with their spiritual health for several reasons. Some people doubt that a higher spirit exists. Other people believe a higher spirit exists, but don't feel worthy of asking for help or don't see the connection between their spiritual health and their mental, emotional, and physical health. Still others believe a higher spirit exists but have an unhealthy or inaccurate vision of what it means to have strong spiritual health.

Other people struggle with external pressures relating to spiritual health. In many ways, the world discourages spiritual development by enacting laws that don't allow God to be mentioned in schools and discourage people from practicing their spiritual life in public. Even the messages in society that encourage us to believe in God have hardwired us to believe in God, but not obey His teachings. Thus, many people who do believe in God do not make it routine to practice His teachings. Finally, there is also a very strong enemy to the Holy Spirit whose sole job is to steal and destroy the hope that the Holy Spirit provides.

Because I grew up in a dysfunctional, stress-filled home, I know what it's like to be hungry for unconditional love and acceptance that a healthy spiritual life promotes. As a young teen, I was introduced to spiritual practice and have spent decades in intense and regular prayer and meditation. I've experienced the growth, connectedness, and peace that a healthy spiritual life provides and I credit my relationship with God for giving me the strength to make it through my family and financial struggles.

I've also seen the power of a healthy spiritual life in clients throughout the years. For example, a client of mine named Cori struggled for years with an unhealthy diet and exercise life. She tried everything she could think of but couldn't find the strength to stick with healthy eating and exercise habits until one night her daughter came crying into her bedroom because she had a nightmare that Cori had died.

While Cori was comforting her and assuring her that it was only a dream and everything was going to be okay, her young daughter began asking questions about Heaven and God. That conversation caused both Cori and her daughter to feel God's presence and power. Cori's daughter told Cori that she asked Jesus into her heart and felt better. Cori realized that she hadn't been taking care of herself and needed God's help to find the will to do so.

She realized she hadn't been thankful to God for all the good in her life. She had been focused on her struggles and mentally and emotionally trying to overcome her struggles on her own with little success. She took a different approach after that conversation with her daughter and reached out to God through prayer and meditation, asking Him to give her the desire, strength, and will to eat healthfully and exercise. She also prayed that God give her family the desire, strength, and will to eat better and exercise together.

That night, she prayed with her family at the table for better health habits. In doing so, she felt stronger because she asked God and got her family involved to ask God for help and for the desire to be healthier.

After years of struggling to do it all herself and finding she didn't have the will to do so, she was finally able to feel the desire and build healthy momentum by working on her spiritual health and accepting the strength of her spirit.

Cori struggled with her body and soul. She was unhealthy and heartsick until she added spiritual focus and practice. After her daughter's nightmare, she was able to gain control of the other two parts of her being. In just a few months, Cori began feeling the effects of a healthier spiritual life. She felt more balanced and in control. She felt physically, emotionally, and mentally stronger. She felt motivated and focused. Cori credits those effects to prayer and spiritual meditation.

Cori's experience, while anecdotal, is supported by several studies on the effect of prayer and meditation on people's overall health, which suggest a link between prayer or meditation and several improved physical and emotional conditions, such as blood pressure, irritable bowel syndrome, anxiety, depression, and insomnia.[64] The Mayo Clinic, for example, indicated that research supports utilizing meditation as a possible way to help people manage symptoms of conditions such as anxiety disorders, asthma, cancer, depression, heart disease, high blood pressure, pain, and sleep problems.[65]

"And he shall be like a tree planted by the rivers of water, that brings forth its fruit in its season; his leaf also shall not wither; and whatsoever he does shall prosper."

Psalms 1:3
King James 2000 Bible

Not only can prayer be a curative tool in times of crisis, but it can also provide a sustained state of well-being. Researchers from Virginia Commonwealth University in Richmond who analyzed 1,900 sets of twins found that twins committed to spiritual lives tended to have lower rates of depression, addiction, and divorce. They also found that the active involvement in a spiritual community was strongly linked to their overall stability and health. Overall, being a part of a body of believers, in addition to prayer, led to better overall stability and health.

Neuroscientist and author of *How God Changes Your Brain: Breakthrough Findings from a Leading Neuroscientist*, Andrew Newberg, has studied the effect of prayer on the human body for over twenty years by injecting radioactive dye into patients and watching changes in their heads when they pray. In addition to his studies, Newberg analyzed over a decade of studies and information on prayer and meditation with his coauthor and concluded that regular prayer and spiritual practice reduce stress, anxiety, and depression—and even slow the aging process. Intense prayer and meditation, they discovered, actually change numerous structures and functions of your brain permanently, strengthening your brain and improving cognitive functioning.

There's more to your spiritual health than just prayer and meditation, although there are proven benefits of both on your three-part being.

Certain factors affect how powerful the benefits of prayer will be. These factors are basically qualities of human consciousness like caring, compassion, empathy, and love. The stronger these qualities are in our lives, the greater the benefits of prayer. That means that if you add these qualities to your consciousness, if you add them to your soul, then the qualities of your soul that we talked about in the last chapter, when combined with a healthy prayer and meditation practice, work together to give health and healing to the third part of our selves: our body.

"He is like a tree planted by water,
that sends out its roots by the stream,
and does not fear when heat comes,
for its leaves remain green,
and is not anxious in the year of drought,
for it does not cease to bear fruit."
— Jeremiah 17:8 (ESV)

You can experience the same spiritual power as Cori and I did by intentionally focusing on exercising a healthy spiritual health plan like the one I show you in this chapter. By doing so, you'll experience better physical and emotional health, more self-love, and a true three-part balance that only a healthy spiritual practice can provide. Without it, you will struggle like millions of others who grow tired of life, feeling everything and everyone is dependent on you and your work. Your emotional life and self-perception will struggle, too. Most of all, you will feel alone and hopeless, and believe life has no meaning or greater purpose than the physical experiences on earth.

This is a proven spiritual health plan.

In Galatians 5:16–18 (NIV), God says, "So I say, walk by the Spirit, and you will not gratify the desires of the flesh. For the flesh desires what is contrary to the Spirit, and the Spirit what is contrary to the flesh. They are in conflict with each other, so that you are not to do whatever you want. But if you are led by the Spirit, you are not under the law." God is telling us in this verse that a healthy spirit will help you overcome unhealthy desires that bodies without spiritual health will succumb to.

You can experience the same strength and power that Cori and I did once we walked closer to God in our struggles by following this simple spiritual plan. This plan will help you unlock the true strength of your will and a power beyond your earthly mental, emotional, and physical capacity.

The first step to improving your spiritual health is to start spending quiet time in meditation with God. For me, this took the form of taking daily walks alone talking to God in my head, and sometimes out loud. I prayed and asked God for the strength and guidance to deal with whatever struggles I had as well as direction to go where I wanted to go.

Second, you need to feed your spiritual self. We feed our bodies through nutrition, exercise, water, sleep, and supplements. We feed our soul through giving, forgiving, and cleansing our hearts of negative thoughts and emotions. It's important that we also feed our spiritual selves, in order to achieve true three-part balance and become healthy, happy, and ultimately, whole.

Because we are three-part beings, comprised of our body, soul, and spirit, we need to practice healthy habits in all three areas to experience true balance

We feed our spirit through prayer and meditation. Psalms 1:2, for example, tells us "But his delight is in the law of the Lord. And in His law he mediates day and night" (NASB). In Psalms 46:10 God tells us to "be still and know that I am God" (NIV). That's what you do when you meditate from a Biblical perspective. You be still and put your thoughts and emotions on God.

Because we are three-part beings, comprised of our body, soul, and spirit, we need to practice healthy habits in all three areas to experience true balance. As you strengthen your spiritual health, you will begin to feel your spiritual life as the final key to unlocking your best health and true happiness, and you'll begin to experience a much healthier, more vibrant, feeling good life.

OPTIMAL LIVING ACTION STEPS

1. Spend five minutes thinking about how you would rate your spiritual health on a scale of 1–10.

2. What changes could you make this week to get closer to a 10?

3. Spend at least five minutes of quiet time in prayer and meditation asking God for strength and direction to improve your body, soul, and spiritual walk.

CHAPTER 8
A NEW BEGINNING

*"It doesn't matter what
your story was or what your story is;
you can start a new story today!"*

– Dr. Phil Carson

YOU MAY HAVE NOTICED that this book doesn't include a conclusion, but instead ends with this Chapter 8. The number eight in the Bible represents a new beginning. Because of that, I decided to end this book with a Chapter 8 that is designed to give you permission and inspiration to move forward with your own new beginning as you build a healthy, happy, and whole life.

> *"Carpe diem! Rejoice while you are alive;*
> *enjoy the day; live life to the fullest;*
> *make the most of what you have.*
> *It is later than you think."*
>
> **– Horace**

No matter what your past looks like or what limitations you face, you can start from right where you are and become happy, healthy, and whole by implementing a simple plan to improve each of the seven N.E.W.S.S.S.S. key areas of your life. These seven key areas can work together to help you achieve better mental, emotional, and physical health in a way that's flexible enough to fit into any budget or lifestyle. They give you everything you need to:

- eat clean and healthfully to avoid unhealthy toxins and processed foods;
- incorporate exercise into your day;
- drink enough good water to ensure that your body stays hydrated and healthy;

- get the right amount and quality of sleep for mental and physical health, energy, and growth;
- identify vitamins and minerals your body needs and how to choose supplements to get you everything you need without any of the unhealthy toxins found in many supplements;
- find mental and emotional peace to cleanse your heart and soul of the heaviness and pain of your past and leave it full of peace and love; and
- develop a healthy spiritual life to give you strength, healing, and the will to implement and stick with healthy habits.

These key areas of life will help you reduce stress, enhance business and personal relationships, and live a healthy, vibrant, feeling good life with more control over your health, wealth, and well-being than you ever imagined.

The next several weeks can be the most important and transformational of your life. They can change your family tree. *You* can change your family tree, but you don't have to do it alone. With the power of a more focused spiritual walk and the information you're now armed with from this book, you have all you need to start. Don't get stuck on your past. Instead, focus on your new beginning toward a healthy, happy, and whole life.

As you begin to work on transforming your body, soul, and spiritual life, I want you to remove three words from your vocabulary. These three words can make the difference between becoming happy, healthy, and whole; or getting stuck in a painful, unhealthy, depressed cycle. By removing them from your vocabulary, you will put yourself in a position to accomplish far more for your health than you ever thought possible.

These words are "can't," "won't," and "don't." These words stop people in their tracks and cause hopelessness and inaction. They create a poisonous mindset and lead to you thinking you can't improve your body, soul, and spirit. They trap your thoughts and words and lead you to tell yourself that you *would* improve your health if you *could*. *Would if I could* thinking reinforces the idea that you *can't* do something, when the reality is that you absolutely *can* improve your health.

Choose to make today your new beginning.

So never say "I can't" because can't never could accomplish anything. Never say "I won't" because won't never will accomplish anything. Never say "I don't" because don't never did accomplish anything.

Instead, I want you to shift your words and mindset into thinking about what you *can* and *will* accomplish. By saying "Yes I can" and "Yes I will," before long you'll be able to proudly say (and celebrate) everything you *did*.

After removing "can't," "won't," and "don't," I want you to also reverse any "would if I could" thinking you may be doing by changing your words into an "I could if I would" sentence that concludes by stating one action you can take to improve your body, soul, and spirit. For example, instead of "I would drink more water if I could get used to the taste," say, "I could drink more water if I would replace one soda with a bottle of water." Realize that you *could* have more peace with your soul if you *would* forgive people who have wronged you. Finally, be confident that you *could* feel more connected to God if you *would* pray daily.

Writing your own "I could if I would" sentences for each of the seven N.E.W.S.S.S.S. key areas of your life with one next step forward for each is your Optimal Living Action Step for your very own new beginning as you finish reading this book. So stop saying you *would* if you *could* and start saying and writing out all the things you *could* do if you *would* take the next positive step.

> "Deem every day of your life
> as a leaf in your history."
> **– Anonymous**

You have far more control of your future health and well-being than you may realize. You hold the keys. There's no reason that you can't work with your family, friends, health-care providers, and spiritual community to start improving each of the seven N.E.W.S.S.S.S. key areas of your life. All you need to do is take the next step. Sometimes that means starting to do something you don't necessarily want to do, but which you know will lead you to a better tomorrow. In the words of the great motivator, Andy Andrews, "The question is . . . can you do something you don't necessarily want to do in order to obtain a result you would like to have?"

Don't get stuck on your past. Instead, focus on your new beginning toward a healthy, happy, and whole life.

I'll leave you today with the same message I use to close my podcast, *The Feeling Good Podcast*, each week, which is to "get out there and *really* live." This is because I believe people who are living out their calling through their body, soul, and spirit aren't just living, but *really* living as God wants us to live. That's what I've built for myself, and what I want for you, too. I want you to experience *really* living as God wants you to live and set the example for others to follow, so they can learn to *really* live as well.

As a follower of Christ, I believe it's my responsibility to *really* live as God wants me to. I also believe it's my responsibility to set an example for my family, especially, but also for others who watch my life. That feeling of responsibility has caused me to live with more passion about my total health, including my body, soul, and spirit.

I want you to have that same passion for your total health, too. I want you to be passionate about living a healthier life because your life matters; you matter. You matter even more to the people you influence and the people you love. When you live a healthy and vibrant, feeling good life, you can live better and maybe even longer. That means you can matter more to those around you, and maybe even over a longer period of time.

We have no idea how many days we are blessed with on earth. We may get only 40, 70, 90, or even 105 years; however, the quantity of those days isn't as important as the quality of life we can have in the days we get. We can all influence that quality by taking care of our body, soul, and spirit we are gifted with.

"Living well is the best revenge."
– George Herbert

If you have any questions about your specific situation or want additional help from me, reach out to me at HowToLiveUntilYouDie.com and I'd be honored to speak with you. You can also sign up for daily inspiration and information that helps you walk through the seven N.E.W.S.S.S.S. key areas and implement them in your life at HowToLiveUntilYouDie.com.

Today can be anything you choose it to be, because you have all the tools you need to change your life. Choose to make it the day you begin to change your life by improving your body, soul, and spirit. Choose to make today your new beginning.

You don't have to go at it alone. Join a group or ask a friend or relative to help keep you accountable. Have regular conversations with your doctors or other health-care providers. If you can afford it, hire a coach, trainer, consultant, or counselor to help you work on your body, soul, and spirit.

I also highly encourage you to join your local church or other place of worship because, as the Scriptures tell us in Phillipians 4:13, you can do all things through Christ who gives you strength.

It doesn't matter what your situation is or how deficient you are in the N.E.W.S.S.S.S. key areas of life, you can start today with your very own new beginning and build a life that is happy, healthy, and whole. You could even be deficient in *all* seven key areas, like Sam, the young man I talked about earlier in the book. Sam pulled himself up from a life of stress, instability, and unhealthy influences by working intentionally over time to improve his body, soul, and spiritual life.

Today, Sam's one of the most healthy, happy, and whole people you will ever meet.

If he can do it, so can you.

I know, because I'm Sam.

I'll leave you with the same Scripture and prayer I offered at the beginning of this book:

"Dear friend, I pray that you may enjoy good health and that all may go well with you, even as your soul is getting along well."

3 John 1:2 (NIV)

CONNECT

CarsonNatural.com

LinkedIn.com/carsonphillip

Twitter: @DrPhilCarsonRx

Facebook.com/carsonnatural

ENDNOTES

1. http://www.health.harvard.edu/healthbeat/ how-stress-can-make-us-overeat

2. http://www.cdc.gov/nchs/data/hus/hus15.pdf#053

3. https://www.nhlbi.nih.gov/health/health-topics/topics/obe/risks

4. https://www.consumer.ftc.gov/topics/weight-loss-fitness

5. https://www.consumer.ftc.gov/articles/0261-dietary-supplements#su pplementsclaimingtobecures

6. http://www.ncbi.nlm.nih.gov/pubmed/20338278

7. http://www.ncbi.nlm.nih.gov/pubmed/15639678

8. http://www.cnn.com/2014/02/10/health/chemical-food-additives/

9. http://jco.ascopubs.org/content/22/2/383.1.full.pdf+html

10. http://jco.ascopubs.org/content/22/2/383.1.full.pdf+html

11. http://jco.ascopubs.org/content/22/2/383.1.full.pdf+html

12. http://today.uconn.edu/2012/02/ even-mild-dehydration-can-alter-mood/

13. https://www.ncbi.nlm.nih.gov/pmc/articles/PMC2908954/

14. https://www.ncbi.nlm.nih.gov/pmc/articles/PMC2908954/

15. https://www.epa.gov/sites/production/files/2015-11/ documents/2005_11_17_faq_fs_healthseries_filtration.pdf

16. http://www.scientificamerican.com/article/ unregulated-chemicals-found-in-drinking-water/

17. http://www.scientificamerican.com/article/ unregulated-chemicals-found-in-drinking-water/

18. http://www.scientificamerican.com/article/ unregulated-chemicals-found-in-drinking-water/

19. http://www.scientificamerican.com/article/ unregulated-chemicals-found-in-drinking-water/

20. http://pubs.acs.org/doi/ipdf/10.1021/acs.estlett.6b00260

21. http://www.ewg.org/research/chromium-six-found-in-us-tap-water

22. https://www.indiegogo.com/projects/ the-right-cup-trick-your-brain-drink-more-water-health-technology#/

23. https://www.ncbi.nlm.nih.gov/pmc/articles/PMC3195546/

24. https://www.ncbi.nlm.nih.gov/pmc/articles/PMC3195546/#sec9title

25. https://health.clevelandclinic.org/2013/10/ what-the-color-of-your-urine-says-about-you-infographic/

26. http://classics.mit.edu/Aristotle/sleep.html

27. http://www.cdc.gov/media/releases/2016/p0215-enough-sleep.html

28. http://www.cbsnews.com/news/
consumer-reports-investigation-sleeping-aids-remedies/

29. http://www.cbsnews.com/news/
consumer-reports-investigation-sleeping-aids-remedies/

30. https://sleep.org/articles/ways-technology-affects-sleep/

31. http://www.cdc.gov/nchs/data/databriefs/db127.pdf

32. http://www.cbsnews.com/news/
consumer-reports-investigation-sleeping-aids-remedies/

33. http://www.cbsnews.com/news/
consumer-reports-investigation-sleeping-aids-remedies/

34. http://sleepdisorders.sleepfoundation.org/chapter-1-normal-sleep/
the-physiology-of-sleep-obesity-weight/

35. http://thechart.blogs.cnn.com/2012/06/10/
sleepy-brains-drawn-to-junk-food/?hpt=he_c1

36. https://www.ncbi.nlm.nih.gov/pmc/articles/PMC3256323/

37. https://www.cdc.gov/media/releases/2011/a0926_insufficient_sleep.
html

38. https://www.ncbi.nlm.nih.gov/pmc/articles/PMC2656292/

39. http://www.webmd.com/sleep-disorders/features/
diabetes-lack-of-sleep#1

40. https://hbr.org/2006/10/sleep-deficit-the-performance-killer

41. https://www.escardio.org/The-ESC/Press-Office/Press-releases/
Poor-sleep-associated-with-increased-risk-of-heart-attack-and-stroke

42. http://www.journalsleep.org/ViewAbstract.aspx?pid=27780

43. https://www.ncbi.nlm.nih.gov/pmc/articles/PMC3959895/

44. http://econweb.ucsd.edu/~magibson/pdfs/sleep_productivity.pdf

45. http://www.telegraph.co.uk/news/health/news/8555899/Lack-of-
sleep-kills-a-mans-sex-drive-study-concludes.html

46. http://www.health.harvard.edu/blog/
little-sleep-much-affect-memory-201405027136

47. https://sleepfoundation.org/how-sleep-works/
what-happens-when-you-sleep

48. https://sleepfoundation.org/how-sleep-works/
what-happens-when-you-sleep

49. https://sleepfoundation.org/how-sleep-works/
what-happens-when-you-sleep

50. https://sleepfoundation.org/how-sleep-works/
what-happens-when-you-sleep

51. http://www.prnewswire.com/news-releases/expert-panel-recommends-new-sleep-durations-300028815.html

52. http://www.prnewswire.com/news-releases/expert-panel-recommends-new-sleep-durations-300028815.html

53. http://www.prnewswire.com/news-releases/expert-panel-recommends-new-sleep-durations-300028815.html

54. https://www.nigms.nih.gov/Education/Pages/Factsheet_CircadianRhythms.aspx

55. https://sleepfoundation.org/how-sleep-works/what-happens-when-you-sleep

56. http://www.aasmnet.org/articles.aspx?id=926

57. https://sleepfoundation.org/sleep-topics/caffeine-and-sleep

58. http://time.com/3671777/drinking-sleep/

59. http://www.everydayhealth.com/sleep/101/improve-sleep.aspx

60. http://www.forbes.com/sites/travisbradberry/2016/09/13/4-reasons-sleeping-naked-makes-you-healthier-and-wealthier/#59ca39ac1c2d

61. http://www.prnewswire.com/news-releases/national-sleep-survey-pulls-back-the-covers-on-how-we-doze-and-dream-184798691.html

62. http://www.apa.org/helpcenter/stress-facts.pdf

63. http://hpq.sagepub.com/content/21/6/1004.abstract

64. https://nccih.nih.gov/health/meditation/overview.htm

65. http://www.mayoclinic.org/tests-procedures/meditation/in-depth/meditation/art-20045858

HowToLiveUntilYouDie.com

42832300R00111

Made in the USA
Middletown, DE
22 April 2017